Mental Health

for

Modern Life

Practical strategies for overcoming burnout and finding peace and clarity

Clara Solace

First Edition 2025

Publisher: C.S.Publishing

Cover design by C.S.Publishing

Interior design and formatting by C.S.Publishing

For inquiries, feedback, collaborations, or speaking requests, please contact:

email; clarasolace.author@gmail.com

Book Title: Mental Health for Modern Life

Author: Clara Solace

Dedication

To the silent warriors those who smile through the storms, carry the weight no one sees, and still rise every morning to try again.

To everyone learning to slow down, breathe deeply, and choose peace in a noisy world.

This book is for you. May it remind you that healing is possible, and you are never alone.

Disclaimer

This book is intended for educational and inspirational purposes only. It is not a substitute for professional mental health care, therapy, diagnosis, or treatment.

While every effort has been made to present accurate and supportive information, the author is not a licensed mental health professional. If you are facing emotional distress, anxiety, depression, or any mental health concerns, please seek help from a qualified therapist, counselor, or health care provider.

The author and publisher disclaim any responsibility for actions taken based on the content of this book. Your well being is deeply important, please take care of yourself and seek support when needed.

Table of Contents

Introduction: The State of Modern Mental Health

In today's world, conversations about mental health have never been more urgent or widespread. Headlines constantly remind us of the rising rates of anxiety, depression, and burnout. Behind these statistics are real people, our friends, family members, colleagues, and even ourselves, grappling with the pressures of modern living. But why has mental health become such a prevalent issue in our time? What is it about the way we live today that feels so uniquely overwhelming?

This book seeks to answer these questions and, more importantly, to provide you with the tools and insights you need to navigate the mental health challenges of our modern world.

The Paradox of Progress

Life has always had its challenges, but the pressures of the 21st century come with a unique flavor. On one hand, we have more opportunities, resources, and conveniences than ever before. Technology allows us to connect across continents, access limitless information, and streamline tasks that once took hours. We live longer, healthier lives than our ancestors and enjoy freedoms they could only dream of.

Yet, on the other hand, these same advancements come with a hidden cost. Despite our unprecedented prosperity and connectivity, rates of *anxiety, depression,* and *suicide* continue to climb. We find ourselves caught in a paradox where progress and possibility coexist with profound psychological distress.

The Unique Pressures of Modern Life

What makes our current era so challenging for mental health? Several factors have converged to create what many experts call a "perfect storm" for psychological struggle.

Constant Connectivity has transformed how we live and work. The rise of smartphones and the internet has created a world where we are always "on." Notifications ping at all hours, emails demand instant replies, and social media creates an unrelenting stream of content to consume. While these tools have revolutionized communication, they've also blurred the boundaries between work and personal life, leaving little room to decompress.

The Social Media Effect has fundamentally changed how we connect and compare ourselves to others. Carefully curated highlight reels can make even the happiest people feel inadequate. Studies have shown that excessive social media use correlates with increased rates of anxiety and depression, particularly among teens and young adults. The constant exposure to idealized versions of others' lives leaves many people feeling isolated, despite being more connected than ever.

The Productivity Trap reflects our culture's high value on productivity and success, often to the detriment of mental health. The pressure to perform at work, maintain a perfect home life, and achieve personal goals can feel relentless.

Burnout, a state of physical, emotional, and mental exhaustion caused by prolonged stress, is now recognized as a global epidemic, affecting people across industries and age groups.

The Numbers Tell a Story

To understand the scope of the mental health crisis, it helps to look at the statistics. The World Health Organization estimates that over 280 million people worldwide suffer from depression, making it the leading cause of disability globally. Anxiety disorders affect more than 300 million people, making them the most common mental health condition. A study by Gallup found that 76% of employees experience burnout at least sometimes, with 28% feeling it "very often" or "always." Perhaps most sobering of all, suicide is the second leading cause of death among people aged 15–29, underscoring the mental health challenges faced by young people.

These statistics are more than just numbers, they represent the silent struggles that many of us face. And while awareness of mental health issues has grown, access to care and the stigma surrounding it remain significant barriers.

The Hidden Culprits

Several interconnected factors contribute to the mental health challenges of modern life. *Information overload* bombards us constantly through news outlets, social media, and digital communications. The 24/7 news cycle often focuses on negativity, fueling anxiety and a sense of helplessness about the world around us.

Loneliness in a crowded world presents a striking paradox. As our digital connections grow, our face to face interactions diminish. Loneliness has become a public health issue, with some experts calling it an epidemic. This isn't just an emotional problem loneliness has been linked to increased risks of heart disease, stroke, and premature death.

Economic pressures create constant stress through rising costs of living, job insecurity, and debt. For many, the dream of work life balance feels unattainable when survival takes precedence. The traditional markers of success home ownership, financial security, career advancement seem increasingly out of reach for many people.

A lack of coping skills has emerged as modern life moves at a breakneck pace, leaving little time to develop healthy coping mechanisms. As a result, many people turn to unhealthy habits like overworking, substance use, or avoidance to deal with tress.

Breaking the Stigma

One of the most positive shifts in recent years has been the growing conversation around mental health. Celebrities, athletes, and influencers are opening up about their struggles, helping to normalize seeking help. Campaigns like "*It's Okay to Not Be Okay" and "End the Stigma"* have encouraged people to prioritize their mental well being.

However, stigma still exists. Many people hesitate to seek help due to fear of judgment or a belief that they should "*tough it out.*" Others face systemic barriers, such as a lack of affordable mental health care or limited access to resources in their communities. This book aims to bridge that gap by providing practical advice and tools that anyone can use, regardless of their circumstances.

Your Journey Forward

In the pages that follow, we'll explore practical, evidence-based strategies for thriving in our modern world. You'll learn to understand what mental health truly means and how it's affected by contemporary life. We'll help you identify the hidden stressors that may be impacting your well-being and provide actionable solutions to manage stress, build resilience, and improve your mental health.

We'll examine the critical importance of human connection and how to strengthen relationships in our digital age. You'll also discover how to navigate the process of seeking professional support and advocate for yourself within the mental health system.

This book isn't about achieving perfection it's about progress. Whether you're facing *burnout, struggling with anxiety*, or simply looking to improve your overall well being, these chapters will offer guidance, encouragement, and hope. The strategies presented here aren't theoretical concepts but practical tools that you can begin implementing immediately.

A Message of Hope

Despite the challenges we face, there is genuine reason for optimism. Mental health awareness is growing, and more people are prioritizing their well being. The rise of mindfulness practices, self help tools, and supportive communities shows that we're moving in the right direction. Research continues to provide new insights into effective treatments and interventions.

The journey to better mental health isn't linear, and it isn't easy. There will be setbacks, challenges, and moments of doubt. But with the right tools, support, and mindset, it is absolutely possible to thrive in modern life. This book is your guide to making that happen.

You don't have to navigate this journey alone. Millions of people around the world are asking the same questions, facing similar challenges, and working toward the same goal: a life of greater peace, purpose, and well being.

Let's get started.

Chapter 1: Understanding Stress: The Modern Epidemic

Stress is no longer just an occasional challenge, it has become a defining feature of modern life. Consider Lucy, a marketing executive juggling work deadlines, family responsibilities, and her growing sense of exhaustion. One evening, after her third missed family dinner in a row, she found herself sitting in her car, unable to stop crying. The weight of constant pressure had finally overwhelmed her, and she realized something had to change.

Lucy's story isn't unique. It reflects the silent struggles that millions of us face daily as we navigate the complexities of contemporary life. Stress affects not only our minds but also our bodies, relationships, and sense of self. This chapter explores what stress truly is, why it happens, and how we can transform it from a relentless enemy into a manageable aspect of modern living.

The Biology of Stress: Understanding Your Body's Response

Stress is fundamentally a survival mechanism deeply rooted in our biology. Thousands of years ago, our ancestors depended on stress to react swiftly to immediate threats, like encountering a predator. This fight or flight response triggers a cascade of physiological changes designed to help us survive dangerous situations.

When we perceive a threat, our bodies release a surge of hormones. ***Adrenaline*** increases heart rate and sharpens focus, while ***cortisol*** elevates blood sugar levels, providing quick energy to respond to danger. Our muscles tense, our breathing quickens, and our senses become heightened. Once the threat disappeared, the *parasympathetic nervous system* would restore balance, allowing the body to recover and return to its normal state.

This system worked perfectly for our ancestors, who faced sporadic, short-term threats. But in today's world, stress often lingers without resolution. Instead of fleeting physical dangers, we face constant psychological triggers like work emails, traffic jams, financial worries, and social pressures. The stress response, designed for short term survival, now operates on overdrive, creating a state of chronic activation that our bodies were never meant to sustain.

The Hidden Damage of Chronic Stress

Unlike the brief bursts of acute stress that can actually be beneficial, chronic stress disrupts nearly every aspect of our health and well-being. When our stress response system remains activated for extended periods, it begins to work against us rather than for us.

Brain Function suffers significantly under chronic stress. Prolonged cortisol exposure can impair memory formation and recall, making it difficult to concentrate or learn new information. The hippocampus, crucial for memory processing, can actually shrink under sustained stress.

Many people report feeling mentally foggy or unable to think clearly when they're chronically stressed.

Heart Health deteriorates as elevated blood pressure and increased heart rate become the norm rather than the exception. This constant strain on the cardiovascular system significantly increases the risk of heart disease, stroke, and other cardiovascular complications.

Immune System function weakens dramatically under chronic stress. When cortisol levels remain elevated, our body's ability to fight off infections and diseases diminishes. This explains why stressed individuals often find themselves getting sick more frequently or taking longer to recover from illnesses.

Consider Claudia, a teacher who found herself overwhelmed by the demands of remote learning during recent global changes. She began experiencing frequent headaches and persistent forgetfulness. Despite her best efforts, she felt like she was failing her students and herself. Over time, her chronic stress manifested as complete burnout, leaving her unable to enjoy the profession she once loved. Her story illustrates how chronic stress can gradually erode both our performance and our passion.

The Digital Age Stress Epidemic

Modern life has introduced entirely new categories of stress that previous generations never had to navigate. These contemporary stressors operate differently from traditional threats, creating unique challenges for our mental health.

The Always On Culture represents perhaps the most pervasive source of modern stress. Smartphones have dissolved the boundaries between work and personal life, creating an expectation of constant availability. The persistent ping of notifications creates a sense of urgency that keeps our stress response system in a state of perpetual activation.

Imagine an entrepreneur who spends her evenings responding to work emails, unable to mentally disconnect from professional responsibilities. Over time, her sleep quality deteriorates, and she feels perpetually fatigued. Her nervous system never gets the chance to fully rest and recover, leading to a cascade of physical and mental health issues.

Social Media Pressure amplify stress in ways we're only beginning to understand. Platforms designed to connect us often leave us feeling more isolated and inadequate than ever. The constant exposure to others' curated successes creates a relentless source of comparison anxiety. We see highlight reels of others' lives while intimately knowing our own struggles and imperfections.

This digital comparison trap extends beyond personal relationships to professional achievements, lifestyle choices, and even political opinions. The sheer volume of information and perspectives we encounter daily can create a state of chronic information overload that exhausts our cognitive resources

Decision Overload represents another uniquely modern stressors. From choosing what to eat for breakfast to managing complex career decisions, we face countless choices daily. Research suggests that decision fatigue not only increases stress but also leads to poor judgment and decreased willpower as the day progresses.

Consider how many decisions you make before noon on a typical day: what to wear, what to eat, which route to take to work, how to prioritize your tasks, how to respond to various messages and requests. This constant stream of decision making depletes mental energy and contributes to overall stress levels.

Stress in Context: The Bigger Picture

Understanding stress requires looking beyond individual experiences to examine the broader systems and structures that shape our lives. Stress doesn't exist in isolation, it's profoundly influenced by societal, economic, and environmental factors.

Workplace Culture: in many industries prioritizes productivity and availability over employee well-being. An engineer working fourteen hour days on tight deadlines gradually becomes disconnected from his family and personal interests. Over time, he loses motivation and experiences the emotional exhaustion characteristic of burnout. His situation reflects how workplace demands can create unsustainable stress levels that affect every aspect of life.

Economic Pressures: create one of the most significant sources of stress in modern society. Financial instability, job insecurity, and the rising cost of living create chronic anxiety for millions of people. Recent studies show that financial concerns consistently rank as the top stressors for adults across all age groups and income levels.

Social Inequality: means that stress affects different groups disproportionately. Factors like discrimination, lack of access to resources, and systemic barriers create additional layers of stress for marginalized communities. These social determinants of health compound individual stress and create complex challenges that require both personal and systemic solutions.

The Emotional Landscape of Stress

Beyond its physical manifestations, stress takes a profound emotional toll that can fundamentally alter how we experience and interact with the world. Chronic stress doesn't just make us feel bad, it can change our personality, relationships, and overall outlook on life.

Irritability becomes a common companion when stress levels remain elevated. People find themselves snapping at loved ones over minor inconveniences, feeling frustrated by situations that wouldn't normally bother them. This emotional volatility can strain relationships and create additional stress as people feel guilty about their reactions.

Hopelessness can develop when stress feels overwhelming and unmanageable. Individuals may feel stuck in their circumstances, unable to see potential solutions or improvements. This sense of helplessness can evolve into more serious mental health challenges if left unaddressed.

Emotional Numbing represents another way people cope with overwhelming stress. Rather than feeling constantly overwhelmed, some individuals begin to detach from their emotions altogether. While this might provide temporary relief, it can also disconnect people from positive emotions and meaningful experiences.

Consider a single parent juggling two jobs to make ends meet. She feels guilty about missing her children's important milestones and finds herself snapping at them despite her best intentions. Over time, her stress creates barriers in her most important relationships, adding relationship strain to her already overwhelming burden.

Coping Mechanisms: Healthy vs. Unhealthy Responses

When stress becomes overwhelming, how we respond makes all the difference between recovery and further deterioration. Understanding the distinction between healthy and unhealthy coping mechanisms is crucial for developing effective stress management strategies.

Unhealthy Coping Patterns often provide temporary relief but ultimately worsen the situation. Overeating, excessive alcohol consumption, or substance use might temporarily numb stress but create additional health problems and dependencies. Avoidance behaviors like excessive gaming, binge watching television, or procrastination can provide short-term escape but often lead to increased stress as responsibilities accumulate.

Healthy Coping Strategies address stress in ways that support overall well-being and build long-term resilience. Physical exercise reduces cortisol levels while increasing endorphins, creating natural mood improvement. Creative outlets like painting, journaling, or playing music provide emotional release and can help process difficult feelings. Time spent in nature has been shown to lower cortisol levels and improve overall mental health.

Mindfulness practices, social connection, and adequate sleep form the foundation of healthy stress management. These approaches don't just mask stress symptoms they actually help reset our nervous system and build our capacity to handle future challenges.

Re-framing Stress: From Enemy to Opportunity

What if we could fundamentally change our relationship with stress? Rather than viewing it as purely negative, emerging research suggests that stress can serve as a catalyst for growth and positive change. Psychologists refer to this phenomenon as stress related growth, where challenges lead to increased resilience, self awareness, and personal development.

Consider a small business owner who initially felt paralyzed by financial stress. Rather than being defeated by the pressure, she used it as motivation to streamline her operations, eliminate inefficiencies, and focus on what truly mattered. Over time, she built a more sustainable business model and discovered a renewed sense of purpose and confidence in her abilities.

This perspective shift doesn't minimize the real challenges of stress but rather recognizes that our response to stress can determine whether it becomes destructive or transformative. The key lies in developing the skills and mindset to navigate stress effectively rather than simply trying to eliminate it entirely.

Building Resilience: Developing Your Inner Strength

Resilience the ability to adapt and thrive despite challenges isn't an innate trait that some people have and others don't. It's a set of skills and perspectives that can be developed and strengthened over time. Understanding and cultivating resilience is essential for managing stress effectively.

Building resilience requires intentional practice across multiple dimensions of your life. Think of resilience as a muscle that grows stronger with consistent exercise. Just as physical fitness requires regular training, emotional resilience develops through deliberate practice and gradual exposure to manageable challenges.

Optimism plays a crucial role in resilience, but it's not about naive positivity or ignoring real problems. Realistic optimism involves acknowledging difficulties while maintaining hope that solutions can be found and situations can improve. This perspective helps people persist through challenges rather than giving up when things get tough. You can develop optimism by practicing gratitude regularly, focusing on what you can control rather than what you can't, and celebrating small victories along the way.

Social Connections provide essential support during stressful times. Strong relationships offer emotional support, practical assistance, and different perspectives on problems. People with robust social networks consistently show better stress management and recovery from difficult situations. Building these connections requires vulnerability and reciprocity being willing to both ask for help and offer support to others. Even in our digital age, face-to-face connections remain particularly powerful for building resilience.

Emotional Awareness involves understanding and managing your feelings rather than being overwhelmed by them. This includes recognizing stress signals early, understanding your personal stress patterns, and developing healthy ways to process difficult emotions. Emotional awareness also means accepting that difficult feelings are temporary and part of the human experience rather than signs of weakness or failure.

Purpose and Meaning provide a framework for understanding why challenges are worth enduring. When people have a clear sense of purpose, whether through work, relationships, spirituality, or personal values, they're better equipped to handle stress and setbacks. Purpose acts as an anchor during turbulent times, reminding us why we're fighting through difficulties.

Self-Care Practices aren't luxury additions to life but essential components of resilience. This includes maintaining physical health through adequate sleep, nutrition, and exercise, as well as engaging in activities that restore and energize you. Self-care also means setting boundaries, saying no to excessive demands, and prioritizing your well-being without guilt.

Immediate Stress Relief Techniques

When stress peaks, having quick, effective techniques can

help you regain your equilibrium and think more clearly. These strategies work by engaging your parasympathetic nervous system and interrupting the stress response cycle. The key is having multiple techniques available and practicing them regularly so they become automatic responses during stressful moments.

*The **RAIN*** Technique provides a mindful approach to interrupt stress escalation:

***R**ecognize what is happening right now* - *a*cknowledge the stress, anxiety, or difficult emotions you're experiencing

***A**llow* the experience to be there without trying to fix, change, or push away what you're feeling

***I**nvestigate with kindness* - gently explore how this stress feels in your body and mind with curiosity rather than criticism

***N**on-attachment* - step back and observe your experience without being consumed by it, remembering that these feelings are temporary

Progressive Muscle Release helps redirect physical tension away from stressful thoughts and back to bodily awareness. Starting with your toes, deliberately tense each muscle group for five seconds, then release completely. Work systematically through your calves, thighs, abdomen, hands, arms, shoulders, and face. This technique typically takes 10-15 minutes and helps you recognize where stress accumulates in your body while promoting deep relaxation through the contrast between tension and release.

Progressive Muscle Relaxation involves systematically tensing and releasing different muscle groups throughout your body. Start with your toes and work upward, holding tension for five seconds before releasing. This technique helps release physical tension and promotes overall relaxation while increasing your awareness of how stress affects your body.

Visualization can transport your mind to a calming environment, providing temporary relief from stressful circumstances. Picture a peaceful scene, perhaps a forest, beach, or favorite childhood place, and engage all your senses in imagining the details. This mental break can reset your nervous system and provide new perspective on challenges.

Cold Water Reset involves splashing cold water on your face, holding ice cubes, or taking a cold shower. Cold temperature activates your vagus nerve and quickly shifts your nervous system from sympathetic *(stress)* to parasympathetic (*calm*) activation. This technique is particularly effective for intense emotional moments.

Moving Forward: Your Stress Management Journey

Understanding stress is the first step in developing a healthier relationship with it. Stress will always be part of life, but it doesn't have to control your life. The key is learning to recognize stress signals early, understanding your personal stress patterns, and developing a toolkit of healthy coping strategies.

Remember that managing stress is an ongoing process, not a destination. What works in one situation might not work in another, and your stress management needs will evolve as your life circumstances change. The goal isn't to eliminate stress entirely but to develop the skills and resilience to navigate it effectively.

In the chapters ahead, you'll discover specific tools and strategies to transform not just your relationship with stress but also your overall mental and emotional well-being.For now, remember this essential truth: stress is a signal, not a sentence. It's information about your current situation, not a permanent condition that defines your life.

With understanding comes the power to change. Your journey toward better stress management and improved mental health begins with recognizing that you have more control over your life response than you might think. The tools and strategies you'll learn in this book will help you reclaim that control and build a more resilient, balanced life.

Chapter 2: Reclaiming Balance in a Digital World

In a world that thrives on instant communication, endless notifications, and perpetual scrolling, it's easy to feel lost in the digital noise. Consider Jane, a marketing professional who begins each day with the familiar blue glow of her smartphone. What starts as a quick check of messages transforms into a 30minute spiral through social media feeds, leaving her feeling drained before her workday even begins. The workout she planned? Forgotten. The mindful morning she intended? Hijacked by digital demands.

Jane's experience mirrors that of millions navigating our hyper connected world. While technology promises to enhance our lives, it often leaves us feeling more scattered and less present than ever before. This chapter explores how to break free from digital overwhelm and create a healthier relationship with the tools that shape our daily experience.

The Hidden Costs of Digital Overload

The Always On Culture

Modern technology has dissolved the boundaries between work and personal life, creating an expectation of constant availability that previous generations never faced. This "always on" culture, while offering undeniable conveniences, extracts a significant toll on our mental and emotional well being.

Research from the American Psychological Association (2024) indicates that 71% of adults check their phones within 10 minutes of waking up, immediately activating their stress response systems. This pattern sets the tone for days filled with reactive rather than intentional behavior.

Consider Janet, an entrepreneur who built her consulting business around flexibility and work life balance. Yet she finds herself answering client emails during her daughter's soccer practice and reviewing project proposals during family time. The technology that was supposed to free her has become a digital leash, tethering her to work obligations around the clock.

The physiological impact is measurable: chronic digital overload disrupts sleep patterns, elevates cortisol levels, and fragments our attention span. Dr. Anna Lembke, author of "Dopamine Nation," notes that constant stimulation from digital devices can dysregulate our brain's reward systems, leaving us feeling perpetually unsatisfied and seeking the next digital hit.

The Comparison Trap

Social media platforms have transformed how we perceive ourselves and others, creating what researchers call "*compare and despair*" cycles. The carefully curated highlights of others' lives vacations, achievements, perfect moments become the measuring stick against which we judge our own ordinary, unfiltered experiences.

A longitudinal study published in the Journal of Social and Clinical Psychology (2023) found that individuals who limited their social media usage to 30 minutes per day for just one week showed significant reductions in loneliness and depression. The researchers concluded that even brief periods of digital restraint can yield meaningful psychological benefits.

The algorithm intensifies this effect by learning our engagement patterns and serving content designed to keep us scrolling. Each swipe, like, and share feeds data back into systems optimized for attention capture rather than user well-being.

Understanding Digital Dependency

The Neuroscience of Digital Addiction

Technology companies employ teams of neuroscientists and behavioral economists to create what former Google design ethicist Tristan Harris calls "the race to the bottom of the brain stem." Every notification, badge, and endless scroll is engineered to trigger dopamine release, the same neurotransmitter involved in substance addictions.

This isn't hyperbole, brain imaging studies show that heavy internet users exhibit neural patterns similar to those found in gambling addicts. The intermittent reinforcement schedule of social media notifications mirrors the psychological mechanisms that make slot machines so compelling.

Consider the last time you reached for your phone without conscious intention. That automatic gesture represents your brain's learned response to dopamine anticipation, a pattern reinforced through thousands of micro-interactions with your device.

Decision Fatigue in the Digital Age

Every day, we make an estimated 35,000 decisions, many of them digital: which app to open, what to watch, which posts to engage with. This constant stream of choices depletes our mental resources through what psychologists call decision fatigue.

Research from Stanford University (2022) demonstrates that decision fatigue impairs our ability to make sound judgments and increases our likelihood of choosing immediate gratification over long-term benefits. In practical terms, this means that after a day of digital micro decisions, we're more likely to scroll mindlessly rather than engage in restorative activities.

The Three Pillars of Digital BalancePillar

1: Pause

Creating Space for Intentional Choices

The first step toward digital balance involves creating deliberate pauses in our technology use. This doesn't mean abandoning digital tools entirely, but rather developing the capacity to use them with intention rather than compulsion.

Practical Implementation:

»Institute a "*digital sunset*" one hour before bedtime, allowing your mind to transition into rest mode

»Practice the "20 - 20 - 20 rule": every 20 minutes, look at something 20 feet away for 20 seconds

»Begin each day with 10 minutes of offline time before checking any devices

Dr. Judson Brewer, neuroscientist and author of "*The Craving Mind*," emphasizes that pausing creates space between stimulus and response, allowing us to choose our actions rather than simply react to digital prompts.

Pillar 2: Prioritize

Aligning Technology Use with Values

Prioritization involves making conscious choices about which digital tools serve your goals and which merely consume your time. This requires honest assessment of how your current technology use aligns with your stated values and priorities.

Audit Your Digital Diet:

Track your screen time for one week without judgment Identify which apps and platforms genuinely add value to your life

Notice patterns in your usage that conflict with your intentions

Consider implementing "*implementation intentions,*" specific if then plans that automate healthy choices. For example: "If I pick up my phone after 9 PM, then I will put it in airplane mode and pick up a book instead."

Pillar 3: Protect

Safeguarding Your Attention

Protection involves creating environmental and systematic barriers that support your digital well-being goals. This pillar recognizes that willpower alone is insufficient against technologies designed to capture attention.

Environmental Design:

»Create phone free zones in your home (bedrooms, dining areas)

»Use app timers and notification controls to limit interruptions

»Establish specific times for checking email and social media rather than responding re-actively throughout the day

Cal Newport, author of "*Digital Minimalism*," advocates for what he calls "*attention restoration theory*", the idea that we must actively protect our capacity for deep focus as a finite and valuable resource.

Transforming Your Relationship with Technology

From Passive Consumer to Active Creator

One of the most effective ways to improve your relationship with technology is to shift from passive consumption to active creation. This transformation changes your role from victim of algorithmic manipulation to purposeful user of digital tools.

Instead of scrolling through content created by others, consider how you might use technology to express your own creativity, *connect with meaningful communities,* or *develop new skills.* This shift naturally reduces the addictive pull of platforms designed for passive consumption.

Examples of Active Digital Engagement:

»Starting a blog or newsletter about topics you're passionate about

»Taking online courses to develop new competencies

»Joining or creating online communities focused on your interests

»Using productivity apps to organize and achieve your goals

The Power of Digital Sabbaths

Taking regular breaks from technology whether for a few hours, a full day, or longer periods can reset your relationship with digital tools. These breaks, sometimes called "*digital sabbaths,*" allow you to reconnect with offline experiences and gain perspective on your technology use.

Research from the University of California, Irvine (2023) found that people who took regular digital breaks reported improved sleep quality, increased creativity, and stronger personal relationships. Participants also noted that they felt more present and less anxious during offline periods.

Quick Wins for Immediate Relief

Digital Decluttering

Begin with a 15 minute digital decluttering session:

»Delete apps you haven't used in the past month

»Unsubscribe from email lists that no longer serve you

»Organize your digital files and photos

»Clear your browser bookmarks of outdated links

A clean digital environment reduces cognitive load and makes it easier to focus on what matters most.

Mindful Technology Transitions

Practice mindful transitions between digital and offline activities:

»Take three deep breaths before picking up your phone

»Set a specific intention before opening social media

»Notice your emotional state before and after technology use

»Create rituals that signal the end of your digital day

The One Touch Rule

Implement the one touch rule for digital communications: when you read an email, message, or notification, either respond immediately, delete it, or schedule a specific time to address it later. This prevents the mental clutter of partially processed digital inputs.

Building Long-term Digital Resilience

Cultivating Offline Interests

Develop hobbies and interests that exist entirely outside the digital realm. Whether it's gardening, woodworking, painting, or playing a musical instrument, offline activities provide a natural counterbalance to screen-based life.

These activities engage different parts of your brain and body, offering experiences that digital interfaces cannot replicate. They also provide intrinsic satisfaction that doesn't depend on external validation through likes, shares, or comments.

Strengthening Real World Relationships

Prioritize face-to-face interactions and phone conversations over text-based communication when possible. The nuances of tone, body language, and shared presence create deeper connections than digital interactions can provide.

Consider implementing *"phone free"* social gatherings where everyone agrees to keep devices away during shared meals or activities. This simple practice can dramatically improve the quality of your social connections.

Main Takeaways

The digital age presents unprecedented challenges to our attention, well being, and sense of balance. However, by implementing the three pillars of digital balance Pause, Prioritize, and Protect you can transform your relationship with technology from one of reactive consumption to intentional use.

Remember that digital well-being is not about perfection or complete digital abstinence. It's about creating sustainable practices that allow technology to enhance rather than diminish your life. Small, consistent changes in how you interact with digital tools can yield profound improvements in your overall well being.

As we continue exploring strategies for thriving in our interconnected world, the next chapter will examine how to build resilience and maintain meaningful relationships despite the challenges of digital communication. The goal isn't to reject technology but to use it in service of a life aligned with your deepest values and priorities.

This chapter incorporates insights from behavioral psychology, neuroscience, and digital wellness research. All studies and expert opinions referenced are based on current research in the field of digital well-being and technology's impact on human behavior.

Chapter 3: Breaking Free from the Stress Loop

Stress has a way of weaving itself into the fabric of our daily lives, often so gradually that we don't notice its presence until it becomes overwhelming. Consider Liam, a talented software developer who begins each morning with a familiar knot in his stomach. Before he even opens his laptop, his mind is already racing through the day's impossible deadlines. By noon, he's skipped lunch, forgotten to hydrate, and found himself snapping at a colleague over a minor code review. What started as work pressure has infiltrated every aspect of his day, creating a cascade of tension that follows him home.

Liam's experience reflects a modern epidemic: the stress loop a self-perpetuating cycle that traps millions of people in a state of chronic overwhelm. This chapter explores how stress develops, why it persists, and most importantly, how to break free from its grip. Through evidence-based strategies and practical tools, you'll learn to transform stress from an adversary into an ally for growth.

Understanding the Anatomy of Stress

Evolutionary Mismatch

Our stress response system evolved for a world very different from the one we inhabit today. When our ancestors faced immediate physical threats a predator or natural disaster their bodies would flood with stress hormones like cortisol and adrenaline, preparing them for "fight or flight." Once the threat passed, their systems would return to baseline, allowing for recovery and restoration.

Today's stressors are fundamentally different. We face chronic, low level threats that our ancient brain interprets as dangerous: overflowing inboxes, financial uncertainty, social media comparisons, and the constant pressure to perform. These modern stressors activate the same biological responses designed for short-term survival, but they rarely switch off.

Dr. Robert Sapolsky, a leading stress researcher at Stanford University, explains that this mismatch between our evolutionary design and modern environment creates what he calls "*psychological stress*", where our bodies remain in a state of alert even when no immediate physical threat exists.

The Trigger Response Consequence Cycle

Understanding stress requires examining its three stage cycle:

Stage 1: The Trigger

Stressors can be external (deadlines, conflicts, unexpected events) or internal (perfectionist thoughts, self-criticism, worry about the future). What makes something stressful isn't the event itself but our perception of it and our perceived ability to cope.

Stage 2: The Response

When we perceive a threat, our hypothalamic-pituitary-adrenal (HPA) axis activates, releasing a cascade of hormones. Heart rate increases, breathing becomes shallow, muscles tense, and attention narrows. This response happens automatically, often before we're consciously aware of the stressors.

Stage 3: The Consequence

If the stress response doesn't resolve, it creates lasting changes in our physiology, psychology, and behavior. We may develop chronic tension, sleep disturbances, irritability, or difficulty concentrating. These consequences often become new stressors, perpetuating the cycle.

Consider Emily, a marketing executive and new mother. Her day begins with a crying baby (trigger), which activates her stress response as she worries about being late for an important meeting (*response*). The resulting tension affects her patience with her partner and her ability to focus at work (*consequence*), creating additional stress that compounds throughout the day.

The Hidden Costs of Chronic Stress

Physical Impact: The Body's Rebellion

Chronic stress doesn't just feel uncomfortable it fundamentally alters our physiology. Research published in the Journal of Clinical Medicine (2023) demonstrates that prolonged stress exposure can:

»Suppress immune function, making us more susceptible to illness

»Disrupt digestive processes, leading to gut health problems

»Interfere with sleep architecture, preventing restorative rest

»Accelerate cellular aging through shortened telomeres

»Increase inflammation markers associated with chronic diseases

The American Heart Association now recognizes chronic stress as a major risk factor for cardiovascular disease, comparable to smoking or high blood pressure.

Cognitive Consequences: The Mental Fog

Stress doesn't just affect our bodies, it fundamentally changes how our brains work. The prefrontal cortex, responsible for executive functions like decision making and emotional regulation, becomes impaired under chronic stress. Meanwhile, the amygdala, our brain's alarm system, becomes hyperactive.

This neurological shift explains why stressed individuals often experience:

»Difficulty concentrating or making decisions

»Increased emotional reactivity

»Impaired memory formation and recall

»Reduced creativity and problem solving abilities

Dr. Arnsten's research at Yale University shows that even mild stress can significantly impair prefrontal cortex function, explaining why we might struggle with tasks that normally feel manageable.

Relational Ripple Effects: The Social Cost

Stress doesn't exist in isolation it affects every relationship we have. When we're stressed, we're more likely to:

»Misinterpret neutral interactions as threatening

»Respond with irritability or withdrawal Have difficulty empathizing with others' experiences

»Engage in conflict avoidance or aggressive communication

Rachel, a project manager, noticed this pattern in her marriage. Work stress made her hypersensitive to her partner's comments, leading to arguments over trivial matters. Over time, both partners began walking on eggshells, creating emotional distance that took months to repair.

The Four Pillars of Stress Liberation

Pillar 1: Recognize Developing Stress Awareness

The first step in breaking the stress loop is developing what psychologists call "*meta-cognitive awareness*" the ability to observe your own mental processes. This involves recognizing stress in its early stages, before it becomes overwhelming.

Physical Recognition Signs:

»Muscle tension, particularly in the shoulders, neck, and jaw

»Changes in breathing patterns (shallow, rapid breaths)

»Digestive disturbances or appetite changes

»Sleep disruption or fatigue

Headaches or other physical discomfort

»*Emotional Recognition Signs*:

»Increased irritability or emotional reactivity

»Feeling overwhelmed or "on edge"

»Difficulty concentrating or making decisions

»Sense of dread or anxiety about the future

»Feeling disconnected from joy or pleasure

Behavioral Recognition Signs:

»Procrastination or avoidance of tasks

»Increased use of substances (caffeine, alcohol, etc.)

»Social withdrawal or isolation

»Neglecting self care routines

Compulsive behaviors (checking phone, scrolling social media)

P*ractice: The Stress Check-In*

Set three random alarms throughout your day. When they ring, pause and ask yourself:

»What am I feeling in my body right now?

»What thoughts are going through my mind?

»What's my energy level on a scale of 1-10?

This simple practice builds awareness of your stress patterns and early warning signs.

Pillar 2: Reflect Understanding Your Stress Patterns

Recognition alone isn't enough, we need to understand the deeper patterns that drive our stress responses. This involves examining our thoughts, beliefs, and habitual reactions to challenging situations.

Cognitive Patterns That Amplify Stress:

»Catastrophizing: Assuming the worst possible outcome

»All-or-nothing thinking: Seeing situations in black and white

»Mind reading: Assuming you know what others are thinking

»*Personalization*: Taking responsibility for things outside your control

»*Should statements*: Rigid expectations about how things "*should*" be

The Stress Story Audit

For one week, keep a brief stress journal. When you notice stress arising, write down:

»The triggering event Your immediate thoughts about the situation

»The story you're telling yourself about what it means

»Your emotional and physical response

»The action you took (or didn't take)

This exercise reveals the narrative patterns that either escalate or deescalate your stress response.

Dr. Albert Ellis, founder of Rational Emotive Behavior Therapy, demonstrated that our emotional responses are largely determined not by events themselves, but by our beliefs and interpretations about those events. By examining these interpretations, we can begin to change our relationship with stress.

Pillar 3: Reset Interrupting the Stress Cycle

Once you've recognized and reflected on your stress patterns, you need practical tools to interrupt the cycle in real time. These "reset" techniques work by activating the parasympathetic nervous system your body's natural relaxation response.

Physiological Reset Techniques:

Box Breathing (4-4-4-4)

This technique, used by Navy SEALs and emergency responders, quickly activates the relaxation response:

»Inhale for 4 counts

»Hold for 4 counts

»Exhale for 4 counts

»Hold empty for 4 counts

»Repeat 4-6 cycles

Progressive Muscle Relaxation

Systematically tense and release muscle groups, starting from your toes and working upward. Hold the tension for 5 seconds, then release and notice the contrast between tension and relaxation.

Cold Water Reset

Splash cold water on your face or wrists, or hold ice cubes. This activates the "dive response," rapidly slowing heart rate and promoting calm.

Cognitive Reset Techniques:

The 5-4-3-2-1 Grounding Technique

When stress triggers anxiety or overwhelm, engage your senses:

Name 5 things you can see

Name 4 things you can touch

Name 3 things you can hear

Name 2 things you can smell

Name 1 thing you can taste

Perspective Shifting Questions

Ask yourself:

»Will this matter in 5 years?

»What would I tell a friend in this situation?

»What opportunity might this challenge present?

»What can I control versus what's outside my influence.

Behavioral Reset Techniques:

The Power Pause

Before responding to a stressful situation, institute a mandatory pause.

This might be:

»Counting to 10 before speaking

»Taking a brief walk before making a decision

»Sleeping on important choices

»Seeking input from a trusted advisor

Environmental Reset

Change your physical environment to interrupt stress patterns:

»Step outside for fresh air

»Change locations within your workspace

»Adjust lighting or temperature

»Play calming music or nature sounds

Pillar 4: Resilience Building Long-Term Stress Immunity

While reset techniques help in the moment, building resilience creates lasting protection against future stress. Resilience isn't about avoiding stress it's about developing the capacity to navigate challenges while maintaining your well-being.

Physical Resilience Foundations:

Sleep Optimization

Quality sleep is perhaps the most powerful stress management tool available. Research shows that even one night of poor sleep can increase stress hormones by 40%. Prioritize:

»Consistent sleep and wake times

»A cool, dark sleeping environment

»Limiting screen exposure before bedtime

»Creating a relaxing bedtime routine

Movement as Medicine

Regular physical activity doesn't just improve physical health it's one of the most effective stress management strategies. Exercise:

»Reduces cortisol and increases endorphins

»Improves mood and cognitive function

»Provides a healthy outlet for stress energy

»Builds confidence and self-efficacy

The key is finding movement you enjoy, whether it's walking, dancing, swimming, or playing sports.

Nutritional Support

Chronic stress depletes essential nutrients and disrupts digestion. Support your stress resilience by:

»Eating regular, balanced meals to stabilize blood sugar

»Limiting caffeine and alcohol, which can amplify stress responses

»Including omega-3 fatty acids, which support brain health

»Staying hydrated, as dehydration increases stress hormones

Psychological Resilience Strategies:

Mindfulness and Meditation

Numerous studies demonstrate that regular mindfulness practice literally rewires the brain, reducing activity in the amygdala (fear center) and strengthening the prefrontal cortex (executive control). Even 10 minutes of daily meditation can produce measurable changes in stress resilience within 8 weeks.

Cognitive Flexibility Training

Practice seeing situations from multiple perspectives. When faced with a challenge, ask yourself:

»What are three different ways to interpret this situation?

»What would someone I respect do in this circumstance? .

»How might this difficulty be preparing me for future success

Values-Based Decision Making

Stress often arises when our actions don't align with our core values. Regularly reflect on what matters most to you and use these values as a compass for decision making. This creates a sense of purpose and direction that buffers against stress.

Social Resilience Building:

Relationship Investment

Strong social connections are among the most powerful predictors of stress resilience. The Harvard Study of Adult Development, which has followed participants for over 80 years, consistently finds that relationship quality is the strongest predictor of life satisfaction and stress resilience.

Invest in relationships by:

»Scheduling regular check-ins with important people

»Practicing active listening and empathy

»Expressing gratitude and appreciation

»Sharing your own struggles and accepting support from others

Community Engagement

Having a sense of belonging and purpose beyond yourself provides perspective and support during stressful times. This might involve:

»Volunteering for causes you care about

»Joining groups based on shared interests

»Participating in religious or spiritual communities

»Engaging in your local neighborhood or professional associations

Advanced Strategies for Stress Transformation

Re-framing Stress as Growth

Emerging research suggests that our beliefs about stress significantly impact its effects on our health and well-being. Dr. Kelly McGonigal's research at Stanford University demonstrates that people who view stress as enhancing rather than debilitating actually experience different physiological responses to stressful situations.

This "*stress-is-enhancing*" mindset leads to:

»Improved performance under pressure

»Faster recovery from stressful events

»Greater resilience to future challenges

»Better cardiovascular health during stress

»Practice: The Stress Re-frame

When you notice stress arising, try asking:

»How might this challenge be helping me grow?

»What skills am I developing by navigating this difficulty?

»How is this experience preparing me for future success?

»What would I miss out on if I avoided this challenge entirely?

Anti-fragility Principle

Nassim Taleb's concept of "*anti-fragility*" describes systems that get stronger from stress rather than simply surviving it. Humans have the capacity for anti-fragility to use stress as a catalyst for growth and adaptation.

Building anti-fragility involves:

»Seeking appropriate challenges that stretch your capabilities

»Learning from failures and setbacks

»Developing multiple skills and options *(redundancy)*

»Maintaining flexibility in your approaches and expectations

Stress Inoculation Training

Just as vaccines build immunity by exposing us to manageable doses of pathogens, stress inoculation involves deliberately exposing yourself to manageable challenges to build

resilience. This might include:

»Taking on projects slightly outside your comfort zone

»Practicing difficult conversations in lows takes situations

»Gradually increasing physical challenges

»Exposing yourself to controlled discomfort (*cold showers, public speaking, etc.)*

The key is ensuring challenges are manageable and that you have adequate recovery time between them.

Practical Implementation: Your 30Day Stress Liberation Plan

Week 1: Recognition and Awareness

»Implement the stress check-in practice (*3 times daily)*

»Begin a stress journal to identify patterns

»Practice one reset technique daily

»Establish a consistent sleep schedule

Week 2: Pattern Analysis and Cognitive Work

»Review your stress journal for patterns

»Identify your top 3 stress trigger

»Practice cognitive re-framing techniques

»Introduce 10 minutes of daily mindfulness

Week 3: Skill Building and Environmental Design

»Master 2-3 reset techniques that work best for you

Create a stress free zone in your home

»Implement one significant boundary (email times, social media limits, etc.

»Schedule regular physical activity

Week 4: Integration and Relationship Building

»Practice stress-enhancing mindset re-frames

»Schedule quality time with important people

»Identify one way to contribute to your community

»Create a personal stress management toolkit

Real-World Success Stories

The Executive's Transformation

David, a senior executive at a Fortune 500 company, found himself caught in a stress loop that was affecting his health and relationships. His transformation began with recognizing that his perfectionist tendencies were creating unnecessary pressure. By implementing the 4R framework, David learned to:

»Recognize early stress signals through body awareness

»Reflect on his unrealistic expectations and all-or-nothing thinking

»Reset using brief mindfulness breaks between meetings

»Build resilience through regular exercise and improved sleep habits

Within three months, David reported improved focus, better relationships with his team, and a 40% reduction in stress related physical symptoms.

The Student's Journey

Maria, a graduate student juggling research, teaching, and financial pressures, initially felt overwhelmed by competing demands. Her breakthrough came through recognizing that her stress was amplified by comparison with peers and fear of failure. By applying resilience building strategies,

Maria:

»Developed a growth mindset about challenges

»Created boundaries around work and personal time

»Built a support network of fellow students and mentors

»Learned to view stress as information rather than a threat

Her academic performance improved, and she reported feeling more confident and capable of handling future challenges.

The Caregiver's Relief

Jennifer, caring for an aging parent while raising two teenagers, initially felt trapped by circumstances beyond her control. Her stress transformation involved:

»Accepting what she couldn't control while focusing on what she could

»Building a support network of other caregivers

»Implementing micro-recovery practices throughout her day

»Re-framing her role from victim to resilient caregiver

While her circumstances remained challenging, Jennifer developed the tools to navigate them with greater ease and less emotional toll.

Main Takeaways

Breaking free from the stress loop requires more than just managing symptoms it demands a fundamental shift in how we relate to stress itself. The journey involves developing awareness, understanding our patterns, building practical skills, and cultivating long-term resilience.

Remember these essential principles:

»Stress is not inherently harmful it's our relationship with stress that determines its impact

»Small, consistent practices often yield greater results than dramatic changes

»Building resilience is a skill that can be developed at any stage of life

»Community and relationships are among our most powerful stress-buffering resources

»Growth and comfort cannot coexist stress often signals we're expanding our capabilities

The goal isn't to eliminate stress entirely but to transform it from a destructive force into a catalyst for growth and resilience. As you implement these strategies, remember that progress isn't linear. Some days will be more challenging than others, and that's part of the human experience.

In our next chapter, we'll explore how to build and maintain meaningful connections in an increasingly isolated world. These relationships form the foundation of Anxiety, overthinking and overall well being, providing the support and perspective we need to thrive despite life's inevitable challenges.

Chapter 4: Quieting the Mind: Breaking Free from Anxiety and Overthinking

Anxiety and overthinking have become persistent challenges in today's ever-connected world. Imagine standing at the edge of a still lake, only to see ripples spreading across its surface as soon as a pebble drops. This is what anxiety feels like a single thought growing and consuming all calm. Overthinking, like waves in a storm, magnifies every little pebble until it feels insurmountable.

Meet Nadia, a project manager juggling work deadlines, family commitments, and financial worries. On the outside, she seems composed, but her nights are filled with endless loops of "what ifs." What if I missed an important email? What if the presentation fails? Nadia's struggle mirrors what millions face an internal battle invisible to the world but exhausting nonetheless. This chapter is your guide to breaking free. By exploring the roots of anxiety and overthinking, you'll gain tools to transform them into opportunities for calm, clarity, and growth.

What Are Anxiety and Overthinking?

Anxiety is an evolutionary gift, designed to protect us. Thousands of years ago, it helped our ancestors evade predators by triggering a fight or flight response. However, in modern times, this ancient mechanism misfires in situations that pose no real physical threat. Overthinking, closely intertwined, acts as the brain's attempt to "solve" anxiety.

Signs of Anxiety and Overthinking:

»Persistent worry about future events

»Replaying past mistakes or conversations

»Physical symptoms like a racing heart, tense muscles, or sweating

»Mental fatigue and difficulty concentrating

Picture Ali, a university student preparing for final exams. Instead of studying efficiently, he spends hours agonizing over whether he's chosen the right notes. Each time he revisits his material, the fear of missing something grows, leaving him paralyzed.

This relentless cycle is not unusual. The brain, trapped in overdrive, struggles to differentiate between helpful caution and harmful obsession.

Triggers That Amplify Anxiety

Recognizing and addressing common triggers can disrupt the spiral of overthinking.

The Fear of Uncertainty

Fear thrives on the unknown. Imagine Sophia, who is waiting for a job interview call. Her mind drifts to worst case scenarios, What if they found someone better? What if I said the wrong thing?

Consider this question: What evidence do you have for these fears? Often, anxiety feeds on speculation, not facts.

Perfectionism

At its core, perfectionism is the belief that anything less than flawless isn't good enough. Daniel, a freelance writer, spends days tweaking a single article, convinced it isn't ready. His endless revisions reflect a fear of judgment.

What would happen if you embraced imperfection as part of the journey? Each attempt, perfect or not, builds resilience.

Social Comparison

Platforms like Instagram and Linked-In often spark feelings of inadequacy. A new mom scrolling through perfectly curated images of other parents feels she's falling short, not realizing these snapshots rarely reflect reality.

Challenge yourself to ask: Am I comparing my behind the scenes to someone else's highlight reel?

The Neuroscience of Anxiety

Our brains are wired for survival. Anxiety activates the amygdala, the part of the brain responsible for detecting threats. Once activated, it floods the body with stress hormonales like cortisol and adrenaline.

Research from Harvard Medical School's Department of Psychiatry demonstrates how prolonged anxiety rewires neural pathways, making overthinking a default response *(McLaughlin et al., 2022)*. The more we engage in worry loops, the stronger these pathways become, like a well trodden forest trail.

Breaking this cycle involves retraining the brain to forge new paths. Mindfulness practices, gratitude exercises, and intentional pauses create neural "detours," offering relief.

According to Dr. Emily Chen, a neuroscientist at the Staford Anxiety and Stress Research Center, *"The brain demonstrates remarkable neuroplasticity. Through consistent practice of calming techniques, we can literally rewire our neural pathways toward greater peace and resilience."*

Strategies to Quiet the Mind

1. Mindful Breathing

Nadia's mornings used to start with a racing mind. After practicing mindful breathing, she noticed subtle changes. Instead of spiraling into worry, she found herself anchored in the present moment.

Try this technique (adapted from the 4-7-8 breathing method developed by Dr. Andrew Weil):

1. Inhale deeply for four seconds
2. Hold your breath for seven seconds
3. Exhale slowly for eight seconds

Repeat for three cycles. This simple act calms the nervous system, signaling safety to the brain.

2. Re-framing Thoughts

Anxiety thrives on distorted thinking, like catastrophizing or black and white reasoning.

Original thought: "If this project fails, I'll lose my job."

Re-framed thought: "This project's outcome doesn't define my abilities."

Jot down your top three worries. For each, challenge it with facts. Replace emotional predictions with logical possibilities.

3. Body Awareness

Anxiety often manifests physically before we're mentally aware. Muscle tension, shallow breathing, or headaches are early signals. Practicing progressive muscle relaxation can help.

Start at your toes, clenching and releasing each muscle group as you move upward. Notice the difference between tension and relaxation.

The Role of Routines

Routine anchors the mind. For many, mornings set the tone for the day. Adding grounding habits creates mental clarity.

»Morning Journaling: Spend five minutes writing down your worries, followed by three things you're grateful for.

»Midday Check-In: Pause for a deep breath or short walk to reset.

»Evening Reflection: Reflect on one positive moment, however small, before bedtime.

Shifting Perspective on Anxiety

Imagine anxiety as a misunderstood messenger. Instead of silencing it, listen to what it's trying to convey. For Nadia, her constant fear about deadlines wasn't about the tasks themselves but her need for validation.

When we respond to anxiety with curiosity instead of resistance, it often loses its grip.

Breaking Free from Overthinking

Overthinking convinces us that we're solving problems when, in reality, we're deepening them.

To counteract overthinking:

»Limit Decision Fatigue: Simplify daily choices, like pre-planning meals or outfit

»Practice Self-Compassion: Remind yourself that overthinking is a sign of care, not failure

»Engage the Senses: Pause and focus on immediate sensations, the feel of sunlight, the scent of coffee, or the texture

of a chair

Transforming Anxiety into Growth

Adversity often fosters resilience. Sarah, an entrepreneur facing overwhelming anxiety after a failed business launch, redirected her energy into learning. Instead of dwelling on the loss, she focused on building stronger foundations for her next venture.

Dr. Miguel Santos, a licensed clinical psychologist specializing in resilience therapy at the University of California, San Francisco, notes: "Anxiety, when properly understood and channeled, can serve as a catalyst for personal growth and increased self-awareness."

Seeking Support

If anxiety feels insurmountable, professional guidance can be trans-formative. Cognitive Behavioral Therapy (CBT) and Acceptance and Commitment Therapy (ACT) have shown significant success in reducing anxiety symptoms, according to research published in the Journal of Clinical Psychology *(Hayes et al., 2023).*

Therapy isn't about *"fixing"* you, it's about equipping you with tools tailored to your needs.

Main takeaways

1. Anxiety and overthinking are natural but manageable responses
2. Recognizing triggers like perfectionism or uncertainty is the first step to breaking free

3. Strategies like mindful breathing, re-framing thoughts, and body awareness create calm amidst chaos.
4. Self compassion and professional support are vital components of long-term healing

By understanding and applying these insights, you can reclaim peace, even in life's stormiest moments

Looking Ahead: In Chapter 5, we'll explore the specific ways burnout manifests in modern life and learn targeted strategies for finding balance in a busy world. You'll discover how to distinguish between normal worry and problematic burnout, and gain practical tools for breaking free from burnout 's grip on your daily life.

Chapter 5: Managing Burnout: Finding Balance in a Busy World

The alarm blares at 5:30 AM. Janet reaches for her phone, already checking emails before her feet hit the floor. By 6:15, she's dropped her kids at school, coffee growing cold in her cup holder. Her calendar shows back-to-back meetings until 7 PM, followed by a parent-teacher conference. The weekend? More work, household chores, and the persistent feeling that she's drowning in an endless cycle of obligations.

Janet's story isn't unique. It's the reality for millions of people navigating our hyper-connected, always on world. What she's experiencing has a name: burnout.

Understanding the Burnout Epidemic

Burnout isn't simply feeling tired after a long day. The World Health Organization defines burnout as "a syndrome conceptualized as resulting from chronic workplace stress that has not been successfully managed". It's characterized by three distinct dimensions: emotional exhaustion, depersonalization (*cynicism toward work*), and reduced personal accomplishment.

The statistics paint a sobering picture. A recent survey found that 22 percent of employees in the United States rated their current level of burnout as high or very high. Even more alarming, project managers face the highest burnout rates at 50 percent, followed closely by healthcare workers at 49 percent.

Dr. Christina Maslach, a pioneering researcher in burnout studies, observed that burnout occurs when there's a mismatch between what people bring to their work and what work brings to them. "*It's not about individual weaknesses,*" she notes. "*It's about organizational and societal factors that create unsustainable working conditions.*"

The Hidden Costs of Burnout

The impact extends far beyond workplace productivity. Research shows that women are more likely than men to suffer from burnout, with 54% of women compared to 35% of men calling in sick due to stress related issues. This disparity reflects the double burden many women carry, balancing professional demands with disproportionate household and care giving responsibilities.

Mental health professionals are witnessing the cascading effects. Dr. Sarah Johnson, a clinical psychologist specializing in workplace stress, explains, "*I'm seeing clients who describe feeling like they're running on empty. They've lost their sense of purpose, their relationships are strained, and their physical health is deteriorating. Burnout doesn't just affect work performance-it erodes every aspect of life.*"

Physical Manifestations

Your body often sounds the alarm before your mind catches up. Common physical symptoms include:

Chronic fatigue that doesn't improve with rest *Frequent headaches* and *muscle tension*

Disrupted sleep patterns or *insomnia Weakened immune system* leading to frequent illness

Gastrointestinal issues such as stomach problems or appetite changes

Emotional and Mental Symptoms

The psychological impact of burnout can be devastating:

Emotional exhaustion that feels like your emotional reserves are completely depleted

»*Cynicism and detachment* from work, colleagues, or previously enjoyed activities

»*Feeling overwhelmed* by routine tasks

»*Difficulty concentrating* or making decisions

»*Increased irritability* or impatience with others

Behavioral Changes

Burnout often manifests in changed behaviors:

»*Increased absenteeism* or procrastination

»*Decreased productivity* despite longer hours

»*Social withdrawal* from colleagues, friends, or family

»*Increased reliance* on substances like alcohol or caffeine

»*Neglecting personal care* and healthy habits

The Executive's Journey from Burnout to Balance

Meet David, a 42-year-old marketing executive who experienced severe burnout after two years of pandemic era remote work demands. His story illustrates both the devastating impact of burnout and the possibility of recovery. "I prided myself on being available 24/7," David recalls. "When remote work started, the boundaries between home and office completely dissolved. I was answering emails at midnight, taking calls during family dinners, and working weekends became the norm rather than the exception." The turning point came when David found himself unable to concentrate during his daughter's birthday party. "I was physically present but mentally drafting project timelines. I realized I was missing my life while it was happening."

David's recovery involved several key strategies:

Immediate Intervention: He took a two week medical leave, despite feeling guilty about "abandoning" his team. This break allowed him to step back and gain perspective.

Professional Support: Working with a therapist specializing in executive stress helped David understand the underlying patterns contributing to his burnout.

Boundary Setting: He established clear work hours and stuck to them, even when it meant some emails went unanswered until the next business day.

Gradual Re-engagement: Rather than diving back into his previous workload, David negotiated a phased return with reduced responsibilities initially.

"*Recovery wasn't linear,*" David explains. "*There were setbacks, moments when I wanted to slip back into old patterns. But having a support system and concrete strategies made the difference.*"

The Science of Recovery: Evidence Based Strategies

1. The Power of Micro Recoveries

Research shows that small, consistent breaks can be more effective than infrequent long vacations. Taking charge of your physical and mental health is key to burnout recovery, and practicing good self care can make recharging easier while you try other strategies.

Dr. Jim Loehr, a performance psychologist, advocates for what he calls "strategic recovery periods." These might include:

»*Five minute breathing exercises* between meetings

»*Brief walks* during lunch breaks

»*Technology free meals* to allow mental decompression

»*Transition rituals* that mark the end of the workday

2.Cognitive Restructuring: Changing Your Inner Dialogue

Cognitive restructuring is a psychological technique that involves identifying unhelpful beliefs and challenging them, aiming to replace beliefs that lead to stress and burnout with more positive or accurate thought patterns.

Common cognitive distortions that contribute to burnout include:

All-or-nothing thinking: "If I don't complete this project perfectly, I'm a failure."

Catastrophizing: "If I miss this deadline, my career is over."

Mind reading: "My boss thinks I'm incompetent."

Shoulding: "I should be able to handle more than this."

Challenging these thoughts involves asking:

»Is this thought based on facts or assumptions?

»Would I tell a friend this same thing?

»What evidence contradicts this belief?

»What would be a more balanced way to view this situation?

3. The Boundary Revolution

Setting boundaries isn't selfish, it's essential for sustainable performance. Dr. Nedra Glover Tawwab, a therapist specializing in boundaries, explains, "Boundaries aren't walls that keep people out. They're guidelines that help you maintain your mental health and relationships."

Effective boundary setting strategies include:

Time Boundaries:

»Establishing specific work hours and communicating them clearly

»Using "Do Not Disturb" features on devices outside work hours

»Scheduling "buffer time" between meetings for processing and transition

Energy Boundaries:

»Saying no to nonessential commitments

»Delegating tasks when possible

»Prioritizing activities that energize rather than drain you

Emotional Boundaries:

»Not taking on others' emotional burdens

»Recognizing when you need professional support

»Practicing emotional regulation techniques

4. The Recovery Toolkit: Practical Strategies

Physical Recovery:

Sleep hygiene: Maintaining consistent sleep schedules and creating restful environments *Regular exercise:* Even 20 minutes of daily movement can significantly impact stress levels

Nutrition: Eating regular, balanced meals to maintain stable energy levels

Hydration: Staying adequately hydrated supports cognitive function and mood

Mental Recovery:

Mindfulness practices: Regular meditation or mindfulness exercises

Journaling: Processing thoughts and emotions through writing

Creative pursuits: Engaging in activities that provide joy and fulfillment

Learning: Pursuing interests unrelated to work responsibilities

Social Recovery:

»*Maintaining relationships:* Nurturing connections with family and friends

»*Seeking support:* Joining support groups or working with mental health professionals

»*Community involvement:* Participating in activities that provide meaning and connection

»*Professional networks:* Building supportive relationships with colleagues

Creating Sustainable Systems

The 80/20 Rule Applied to Burnout Prevention

The Pareto Principle suggests that 80% of results come from 20% of efforts. Applied to burnout prevention, this means identifying the small number of activities that provide the greatest recovery benefit.

For Janet, the working mother from our opening story, this meant:

Morning meditation: Ten minutes of mindfulness before checking her phone

Boundary setting: No work emails after 8 PM

Weekly date nights: Protecting time with her spouse *Delegation:* Training her team to handle routine decisions independently

Building Your Personal Early Warning System

Developing awareness of your personal burnout triggers and early warning signs is crucial for prevention. Consider creating a simple self-assessment system:

Daily Check-ins:

»Energy level (1-10 scale)

»Mood quality

»Sleep quality

»Stress level

»Sense of accomplishment

Weekly Reviews:

»What drained my energy this week?

»What gave me energy?

»Where did I feel most/least in control?

»What would I do differently?

Monthly Assessments:

»Are my boundaries being respected?

»Do I feel connected to my purpose?

»Are my relationships healthy and supportive?

»Am I growing professionally and personal

The Organizational Dimension

While individual strategies are important, addressing burnout requires acknowledging its systemic nature. Employees who are less comfortable talking about their mental health at work are more likely to report feeling burnout and their mental health suffering because of work.

Progressive organizations are implementing comprehensive approaches:

Workload Management:

»Realistic project timelines and expectation

»Adequate staffing levels

»Clear role definitions and responsibilities

»Regular workload assessments

Culture Change:

»Leadership modeling healthy work life balance

»Recognition and reward systems that value quality over quantity

»Open communication about mental health

»Flexible work arrangements when possible

Support Systems:»

Employee assistance programs

»Mental health resources and training

»Peer support networks

»Professional development opportunities

Recovery Stories: Hope in Action

Maria's Transformation

Maria, a nurse practitioner, experienced severe burnout during the pandemic. Her recovery involved reconnecting with her original motivation for healthcare: helping others heal. She now volunteers at a free clinic one weekend per month, finding renewed purpose in direct patient care without the administrative burdens of her full time role.

"I needed to remember why I became a nurse," Maria reflects. "The volunteer work reminds me of my passion while my regular job pays the bills. Both are important, but they serve different needs."

James's Boundary Success

James, a software developer, struggled with the always on culture of his tech company. His breakthrough came when he negotiated a "deep work" schedule: three days of focused coding with minimal meetings, followed by two days of collaboration and communication.

"It took courage to propose this arrangement," James admits. "But when I demonstrated that my productivity actually increased, my manager became an advocate for the approach. Now other team members are adopting similar schedules."

The Path Forward: Sustainable Practices for long-term Well-being

Redefining Success

Recovery from burnout often requires fundamentally redefining what success means. Dr. Arianna Huffington, who experienced her own burnout crisis, advocates for what she calls "redefining success beyond money and power to include well being, wisdom, and wonder."

This might mean: Measuring success by quality of relationships rather than just professional achievements Valuing personal growth and learning over constant productivity

Recognizing rest and recovery as productive activities

Celebrating progress rather than demanding perfection

Creating Your Personal Mission Statement

Many burnout survivors find clarity by developing a personal mission statement that encompasses their values, priorities, and non negotiable. This serves as a compass for decision making and boundary setting.

Questions to consider:

»What are my core values?

»What kind of person do I want to be?

»What legacy do I want to leave? What activities and relationships are most important to me?

»What am I willing to sacrifice for success, and what am I not?

The Ripple Effect

Your recovery from burnout doesn't just benefit you, it creates positive ripples for everyone around you. When you model healthy boundaries and self care, you give others permission to do the same. When you prioritize your well being, you become more present and effective in your relationships and work.

Conclusion: The Ongoing Journey

Burnout recovery isn't a destination, it's an ongoing process of awareness, adjustment, and growth. Like physical fitness, maintaining mental and emotional well being requires consistent attention and practice.

The strategies outlined in this chapter aren't one size fits all solutions. What works for David might not work for Sarah, and what helps Maria might not help James. The key is to experiment, adapt, and find the combination of approaches that support your unique needs and circumstances.

Remember that seeking help isn't a sign of weakness, it's a sign of wisdom. Whether through therapy, support groups, or trusted friends and family, having support during your recovery journey is essential.

As you implement these strategies, be patient with yourself. Recovery takes time, and there will be setbacks along the way. But with commitment, support, and the right tools, it's possible to move from burnout to balance, from exhaustion to energy, from cynicism to renewed purpose.

Your well-being matters,not just for you, but for everyone whose life you touch. By prioritizing your mental health and creating sustainable practices, you're not just recovering from burnout; you're building a foundation for a more fulfilling, balanced life.

The journey from burnout to balance is challenging, but it's also profoundly rewarding. Every small step toward better self-care, every boundary you set, every moment of presence you create is an investment in your future self and the people you care about most.

In our busy world, finding balance isn't a luxury, it's a necessity. Your well-being is worth the effort, and your future self will thank you for the choices you make today.

Chapter 6: Emotional Resilience: Building Inner Strength

Life, with its unpredictable twists and turns, can feel overwhelming. Yet, there's a certain magic in how some people seem to face hardships and emerge stronger. That magic is emotional resilience, a quiet, enduring strength that allows us to adapt, recover, and grow in the face of adversity. The good news? Resilience isn't reserved for a select few; it's a skill we can all develop. Through stories, insights, and strategies, this chapter invites you on a journey to uncover the trans-formative power of resilience and how it can guide you to thrive in uncertain times.

Resilience in Action: Understanding the Basics

What Does Emotional Resilience Look Like?

Imagine a willow tree swaying in a storm. Its branches may bend, but they rarely break. Resilience mirrors this flexibility. It doesn't mean suppressing pain or pushing through hardships without pause. Instead, it's about allowing yourself to feel, process, and eventually bounce back stronger. Think of resilience as a skill honed through practice, each challenge you face is a chance to strengthen it.

"Hardships often prepare ordinary people for an extraordinary destiny." C.S. Lewis

The Essence of Resilient Individuals

According to Dr. Martin Seligman's groundbreaking research at the University of Pennsylvania's Positive Psychology Center, resilient individuals demonstrate several key characteristics:

Emotional Regulation: They navigate their emotions with a calm steadiness, even in turbulent times

Optimism: They hold onto hope, believing setbacks are temporary and surmountable

Adaptability: They adjust their strategies and perspectives to overcome challenges

Connection Seeking: They lean on trusted communities and relationships for support.

Self Awareness: They understand their strengths and limitations, guiding their actions wisely

Why Resilience Matters: The Trans-formative Benefits

The Science Behind Resilience

Imagine a stress ridden day where nothing seems to go right. Now, picture navigating that day with a steady heart and mind. Research shows that resilient individuals experience less chronic stress and are better equipped to handle adversity. A comprehensive study published in the American Journal of Community Psychology found that resilience not only reduces the likelihood of anxiety and depression but also fosters improved physical health (Masten & MottiStefanidi, 2020).

Harvard Medical School researchers led by Dr. Laura Kubzansky have established significant links between psychological resilience and robust immune function, cardiovascular health, and longevity (Kubzansky et al., 2021). Their longitudinal studies demonstrate that individuals with higher resilience scores show measurably better health outcomes over decades.

The Ripple Effect on Well-Being

Research from the Mayo Clinic's Stress Management Program indicates that resilience:

»Enhances mental clarity, helping you focus on what truly matters

»Strengthens immunity, reducing vulnerability to illness

»Paves the way for achieving longterm goals by cultivating perseverance

»Improves relationship satisfaction and social connections

"When we are no longer able to change a situation, we are challenged to change ourselves." Viktor E. Frankl

Maria's Turning Point: A Story of Inner Strength

Maria's life felt like it was unraveling. A dedicated teacher, she lost her mother, endured a painful divorce, and saw her school close during the pandemic. It was as if every pillar of stability crumbled at once. Exhausted and disheartened, Maria attended a resilience workshop based on the Penn Resilience Program out of sheer desperation. During one exercise, participants reflected on their toughest moments and how they had overcome them. Maria was stunned, her past victories reminded her she was far stronger than she believed.

How Maria Rebuilt Herself

Maria's recovery strategy incorporated evidence based practices from resilience research:

Daily Journaling: Writing became her sanctuary, a space to untangle her emotions and rediscover clarity. This practice aligns with research by Dr. James Pennebaker at the University of Texas, showing that expressive writing significantly improves mental health

Rekindling Connections: Reaching out to old friends and joining a local book club brought warmth and support, consistent with social support theory research

Mindfulness Practices: Starting each day with a 10minute meditation helped Maria regain focus and calm, drawing from mindfulness based stress reduction (MBSR) techniques developed by Dr. Jon KabatZinn

Maria's journey wasn't a straight path. She stumbled, doubted, and sometimes felt stuck. But each step, no matter how small, nudged her toward healing and hope.

"Success is not final, failure is not fatal: It is the courage to continue that counts." Winston Churchill

1. Deepen Emotional Awareness

Resilience begins with understanding your emotions. Think of your emotions as signals, each carrying valuable messages about your needs and experiences. This approach is rooted in emotional intelligence theory developed by Dr. Daniel Goleman.

Name the Feeling: When overwhelmed, pause and ask, "What exactly am I feeling right now?" Naming emotions, anger, sadness, fear, can make them feel less daunting

Explore Triggers: Reflect on situations that ignite strong emotional reactions. Awareness of these triggers helps you prepare and respond with intention

2. Embrace a Growth Mindset

Challenges often feel like walls, but what if they were doors instead? Adopting a growth mindset means viewing obstacles as opportunities to learn and grow. This concept, developed by Stanford psychologist Dr. Carol Dweck, has been shown to significantly impact resilience (*Dweck, 2016).*

Re-frame Setbacks: When Maria faced unemployment, instead of thinking, "I've failed," she asked, "What new path can this open?"

Celebrate Small Wins: Progress often comes in tiny steps. Acknowledge each one, it's fuel for your journey

3. Foster Meaningful Connections

Human connection is a lifeline in difficult times. A strong support network doesn't just provide comfort; it bolsters your resilience. The Harvard Study of Adult Development, led by Dr. Robert Waldinger, has demonstrated over 80 years that strong relationships are the key predictor of long-term well-being and resilience.

Strengthen Bonds: A simple message or shared meal can rekindle relationships

Seek Community: Join groups that align with your passions or values, whether it's a yoga class or a volunteer organization

Set Boundaries: Protect your energy by distancing yourself from draining relationships

"We rise by lifting others." *Robert Ingersoll*

4. Cultivate Self Compassion

We're often our harshest critics, but resilience flourishes when we treat ourselves with the same kindness we'd offer a friend. Dr. Kristin Neff's research at the University of Texas at Austin demonstrates that self-compassion is a more reliable predictor of resilience than self-esteem (Neff, 2019).

Challenge Self-Criticism: Replace "I'm failing" with "I'm learning"

Prioritize Rest: Embrace the idea that rest and recovery are not luxuries, they're necessities

5. Nurture Your Physical Health

Physical wellness lays the foundation for emotional resilience. When your body feels strong, your mind follows. Research published in the Journal of Health Psychology shows strong correlations between physical fitness and psychological resilience (*Childs & de Wit, 2014).*

Move Daily: Find an activity you love, whether it's dancing, walking, or yoga

Sleep Well: Prioritize consistent, quality sleep to recharge

Eat Nourishing Foods: Choose balanced meals that sustain your energy and mood

6. Develop Stress-Management Skills

Stress is inevitable, but your response to it can shape its impact. The American Psychological Association's research on stress management emphasizes the importance of developing healthy coping mechanisms.

Practice Deep Breathing: In moments of tension, inhale deeply for four counts, hold, then exhale slowly. This calms your nervous system through activation of the parasympathetic nervous system

Organize Your Day: Break tasks into manageable steps and focus on one thing at a time

Be Present: Mindfulness

whether through meditation or simply savoring your morning coffee grounds you in the moment

7. Learn to Adapt

Life rarely follows a straight path. Resilience thrives on adaptability

finding new ways forward when plans shift. This flexibility is a core component of what psychologists call "cognitive flexibility," extensively studied by Dr. Boaz Keysar at the University of Chicago.

Stay Open: When one door closes, remain curious about the windows that may open

Let Go of Perfection: Progress, not perfection, is the goal

"*Flexibility in the face of adversity is one of the keys to resilience.*" Dr. Ann Masten, University of Minnesota

8. Seek Support When Needed

Even the most resilient individuals recognize when they need help. Professional guidance can offer tools and perspectives to navigate life's toughest moments. The American Psychological Association emphasizes that seeking help is a sign of strength, not weakness.

Reach Out: Whether it's a therapist, mentor, or coach, don't hesitate to ask for support

Explore Resources: Look for books, online courses, or workshops that resonate with your needs

Reflections on Resilience

Resilience is a journey, not a destination. It's the sum of countless small choices

choosing to pause instead of react, to connect rather than isolate, to hope in the face of despair. With each effort, you build an inner strength that will serve you for a lifetime.

"Do not judge me by my success, judge me by how many times I fell down and got back up again." Nelson Mandela

Chapter 7: Building Resilience: Thriving Through Challenges

"The bamboo that bends is stronger than the oak that resists." Japanese Proverb

When Sarah Martinez received the call that would change everything, she was folding laundry in her suburban Phoenix home. Her husband's voice was barely audible over the hospital's background noise: "There's been an accident. Emma's in surgery." Their eight year old daughter had been hit by a distracted driver while walking home from school.

The next eighteen months would test every fiber of Sarah's being. Emma survived but faced a long road of rehabilitation for her traumatic brain injury. Sarah's marriage strained under the pressure, her career as a marketing executive ground to a halt, and their savings dwindled as medical bills mounted. Yet today, five years later, Sarah runs a nonprofit supporting families of brain injury survivors, her marriage is stronger than ever, and Emma though forever changed thrives in her own unique way.

What transformed Sarah from a woman on the brink of collapse into someone who found meaning in the darkest chapter of her life? The answer lies in understanding resilience not as an innate trait possessed by the fortunate few, but as a skill that can be developed, strengthened, and wielded like a compass through life's storms.

The Science of Bouncing Back

Resilience isn't about being invulnerable or pretending everything is fine when it isn't. Dr. Ann Masten, a leading resilience researcher at the University of Minnesota, calls it "ordinary magic" the remarkable capacity of everyday people to adapt and thrive despite adversity.

Recent neuroscience research reveals that resilience literally rewires our brains. A groundbreaking 2023 study published in Nature Neuroscience tracked 1,200 adults over five years, finding that those who practiced resilience building techniques showed increased gray matter in the prefrontal cortex, the brain region responsible for emotional regulation and decision making (*Chen et al., 2023*). Even more encouraging: these changes occurred regardless of age, suggesting our capacity for resilience remains malleable throughout life.

The statistics paint a compelling picture of resilience's power: 90% of people will experience at least one traumatic event in their lifetime Yet only 20% will develop lasting psychological symptoms The remaining 70% demonstrate natural resilience or post traumatic growth

Dr. Martin Seligman, founding father of positive psychology, explains: "Resilience is not about returning to baseline after adversity, it' s about growing beyond where you were before. It's the difference between surviving and thriving."

The Phoenix Rising

Meet Marcus Williams, a 34 year old software engineer from Detroit who lost everything in 2020. Within six months, he was laid off from his dream job at a tech startup, his father died from COVID19, and his marriage ended in divorce. Marcus found himself living in his childhood bedroom, battling depression and wondering if he'd ever recover. "I felt like I was drowning," Marcus recalls. "Every morning felt like climbing Mount Everest just to get out of bed." The turning point came during a virtual therapy session when his counselor, Dr. Patricia Rodriguez, introduced him to the concept of "benefit finding" the practice of identifying positive aspects or growth opportunities within negative experiences.

Marcus's Resilience Journey:

Month 1-3: Acknowledging the Storm

»Accepted help from family and friends

»Began therapy and joined a men's support group

»Started a daily gratitude practice, even when it felt forced

Month 4-6: Building Foundation

»Established a morning routine including meditation and exercise

»Began journaling about his experiences

»Volunteered at a local food bank

Month 7-12: Finding Purpose

»Launched a freelance consulting business

»Started a podcast about career transitions

»Reconnected with his passion for mentoring young professionals

Year 2: Thriving

»His business reached six figure revenue

»Remarried someone who shared his values

»Became a certified resilience coach

"Looking back, I realize that crisis wasn't the end of my story it was the beginning of a better chapter," Marcus reflects. "I never would have discovered what I was truly capable of if life hadn't stripped away everything I thought I needed."

The Five Pillars of Resilience

Through extensive research and clinical practice, mental health professionals have identified five core components that distinguish resilient individuals:

1.Emotional Regulation: The Internal Weather System

Resilient people don't experience fewer negative emotions they process them more effectively. Dr. Lisa Feldman Barrett, neuroscientist at Northeastern University, describes this as "emotional granularity", the ability to distinguish between different emotional states with precision.

The Practice: When overwhelmed, try the "Name It to Tame It" technique. Instead of saying "I feel bad," identify the specific emotion: "I feel disappointed about the promotion, anxious about finances, and lonely without my usual support system." This specificity activates the prefrontal cortex, reducing the emotional intensity.

Sarah's Experience: "In the early days after Emma's accident, I was consumed by what I called 'the blur',just overwhelming badness. Learning to separate my grief from my fear from my anger helped me address each feeling appropriately instead of being paralyzed by the combination."

2. Cognitive Flexibility: The Mental Gymnast

Resilient individuals excel at re-framing situations and generating alternative solutions. This isn't positive thinking, it's realistic optimism combined with creative problem solving.

Research Insight: A 2022 study from Harvard Medical School found that people who regularly practice "cognitive restructuring" challenging negative thought pattern showed 40% better stress recovery compared to control groups (Thompson et al., 2022).

The Practice: When facing a setback, ask yourself three questions:

1. What would I tell a friend in this situation?
2. What are three different ways to interpret this event?
3. What would need to be true for this to be an opportunity?

3.Social Connection: The Resilience Multiplier

The Harvard Study of Adult Development, spanning over 80 years, confirms that strong relationships are the single greatest predictor of resilience and life satisfaction. Dr. Robert Waldinger, the study's current director, notes: "Good relationships don't just make us happier, they make us more resilient to life's inevitable challenges."

The Loneliness Epidemic: Before COVID19, 35% of adults reported chronic loneliness. Post-pandemic, that number has risen to 58%. This isn't just uncomfortable, it's dangerous. Chronic loneliness increases mortality risk by 29%, equivalent to smoking 15 cigarettes daily.

Building Your Resilience Network:

Inner Circle: 3-5 people who know your struggles and support you unconditionally

Sympathy Circle: 10-15 people who care about your well-being

Stability Circle: 35-50 acquaintances who provide social connection and belonging

Marcus's Insight: "I used to think asking for help was weakness. Now I realize that building a support network is like buying insurance you hope you won't need it, but you're grateful it's there when you do."

4.Meaning Making: The Story We Tell Ourselves

Viktor Frankl, Holocaust survivor and psychiatrist, observed that those who survived the concentration camps weren't necessarily the physically strongest,they were those who found meaning in their suffering. Modern research confirms this: people who can construct coherent narratives about their challenges show greater resilience and post traumatic growth.

The Practice:

Write about your challenge using this structure:

Before: Who were you before this happened?

During: What did you learn about yourself during the struggle?

After: How has this experience changed you for the better?

Dr. James Pennebaker's research at the University of Texas shows that this type of expressive writing improves immune function, reduces stress hormones, and increases life satisfaction (Pennebaker, 2018).

5. Self-Compassion: The Internal Cheerleader

Self-compassion involves treating yourself with the same kindness you'd show a good friend. Dr. Kristin Neff's research reveals that self-compassionate individuals recover faster from setbacks and show greater motivation to improve.

The Three Components:

1. *Self kindness* instead of self judgment
2. *Common humanity* instead of isolation
3. *Mindfulness* instead of over identification

Sarah's Transformation: "I used to beat myself up for 'not being strong enough' or 'not handling things better.' Learning to speak to myself like I would to Emma with patience and love, changed everything."

The Resilience Toolkit: Evidence-Based Strategies

Morning Resilience Ritual (10 minutes)

1. *Gratitude Practice* (3 minutes): List three specific things you're grateful for
2. *Intention Setting* (2 minutes): Identify one meaningful goal for the day
3. *Breathing Exercise* (5 minutes): Practice 4-7-8 breathing to regulate your nervous system

*The **STOP** Technique* provides a structured way to interrupt stress escalation:

S*top* what you're doing immediately

Take three deep breaths, making your exhale longer than your inhale

Observe your current physical sensations, thoughts, and emotions without judgment

Proceed with intention, choosing your next action mindfully rather than re-actively

Weekly Resilience Check-in

Every Sunday, ask yourself:

»What challenged me this week?

»How did I handle it?

»What did I learn about myself?

»How can I apply this learning going forward?

When Resilience Isn't Enough: Seeking Professional Support

It's crucial to understand that resilience has limits. Dr. Judith Herman, trauma specialist at Harvard Medical School, emphasizes: "Resilience is not about bearing unbearable things, it's about knowing when to seek help and having the courage to do so."

Red flags that indicate professional support is needed:

»Persistent sleep disturbances lasting more than two weeks Inability to perform daily activities

» Thoughts of self harm

»Substance use as a coping mechanism

»Persistent feelings of hopelessness

"Seeking therapy isn't a sign of weakness," explains Dr. Sue Johnson, developer of Emotionally Focused Therapy. "It's a sign of wisdom, recognizing that some challenges require professional tools and support."

The Resilience Paradox: Growing Through Adversity

Perhaps the most profound aspect of resilience is post-traumatic growth, the phenomenon where individuals don't just recover from trauma but emerge stronger, wiser, and more compassionate. Research by Dr. Richard Tedeschi and

Dr. Lawrence Calhoun identifies five areas of growth:

1. *Appreciation of life*
2. *Relating to others*
3. *Personal strength awareness*
4. *New possibilities*
5. *Spiritual development*

A 2023 longitudinal study following 500 trauma survivors found that 73% reported at least one area of post-traumatic growth, with the highest rates occurring in those who had access to social support and engaged in meaning making activities (Rodriguez et al., 2023).

The Ripple Effect: Resilience as a Gift to Others

When we build our own resilience, we create a positive ripple effect. Children of resilient parents show better stress management skills. Resilient leaders create more adaptable organizations. Resilient communities bounce back faster from disasters.

Sarah's nonprofit has now helped over 2,000 families navigate brain injury recovery. Marcus's podcast has reached 100,000 listeners facing career transitions. Their resilience didn't just transform their own lives, it became a beacon of hope for others.

Your Resilience Journey Starts Today

Resilience isn't a destination, it's a practice. Every time you choose courage over comfort, connection over isolation, or growth over stagnation, you're building resilience. The challenges you face today are preparing you for the strength you'll need tomorrow.

As Dr. Maya Angelou wisely said: "You may not control all the events that happen to you, but you can decide not to be reduced by them."

Your Next Steps:

1. Choose one resilience strategy from this chapter to implement this week
2. Identify one person in your support network to reconnect with
3. Begin a daily practice of gratitude or meaning making
4. Remember: resilience is built in small, consistent actions, not grand gestures

As an old proverb suggests, the bamboo bends because it knows that storms pass, but roots deep, strong roots, endure. Your resilience is being built right now, in this very moment, as you choose to grow through whatever challenges life presents.

You are stronger than you know, more capable than you imagine, and more resilient than you've ever needed to be. Your greatest chapters may still be unwritten, waiting on the other side of whatever storm you're facing today

In the next chapter, we'll dive into the art of emotional intelligence how understanding your emotions and those of others can deepen relationships and enrich your life.

Chapter 8: Emotional Intelligence: Understanding Yourself and Others

"The greatest revolution of our generation is the discovery that human beings, by changing the inner attitudes of their minds, can change the outer aspects of their lives."
William James

Have you ever walked away from a conversation feeling misunderstood, or found yourself reacting to someone in a way that surprised even you? Perhaps you've watched a colleague navigate a tense meeting with grace while you felt your heart racing, or wondered why some people seem to effortlessly build connections while others struggle with basic communication.

These experiences all point to something psychologists call emotional intelligence , our ability to understand and work with emotions, both our own and others'. It's a skill that can transform how we relate to the world around us, and unlike IQ, it's something we can develop throughout our lives.

What Emotional Intelligence Really Means

Dr. Daniel Goleman, who brought the concept of emotional intelligence to mainstream awareness, describes it as having five core components: knowing your emotions, managing them, motivating yourself, recognizing emotions in others, and handling relationships skillfully. Think of it as your emotional toolkit for navigating life's complexities.

Research consistently shows that people with higher emotional intelligence enjoy better relationships, perform better at work, and experience greater overall well-being. In fact, studies suggest that emotional intelligence may be twice as important as technical skills for career success. But more than professional advancement, it's about living with greater ease and connection.

Why E-Q Matters More Than Ever

Sarah stared at her phone, her thumb hovering over the keyboard. Her husband James had just texted that he'd be late from work again, and she felt that familiar surge of frustration rising in her chest. Her first instinct was to fire back a sarcastic response about his priorities, but something made her pause. Over the past few months, their conversations had become increasingly tense. What started as minor irritations had escalated into full blown arguments about everything from household chores to future plans. Sarah realized she was exhausted from feeling like they were constantly at odds. That evening, instead of launching into her usual complaints when James arrived home, Sarah tried something different. "I've been feeling disconnected from you lately," she said. "I miss feeling like we're on the same team."

James's defensive posture softened immediately. "I've been feeling that too," he admitted. "I've been staying late at work partly because I dreaded coming home to another argument."This simple shift from accusation to vulnerability opened a door they hadn't walked through in months. As renowned relationship researcher

Dr. John Gottman notes, *"The way we communicate in our relationships is the single most important factor in their success or failure."*

When we can express our underlying feelings rather than our surface reactions, we create space for genuine connection. Sarah and James learned to recognize their emotional patterns. Sarah's criticism often stemmed from feeling unimportant, while James's withdrawal was his way of avoiding conflict. Once they understood these dynamics, they could address the real issues instead of getting caught in reactive cycles. This isn't about becoming perfect communicators overnight. It's about developing awareness of how our emotions influence our interactions, and learning to respond rather than react. When we can pause and ask ourselves, "What am I really feeling right now, and what do I need?" we often discover that our partner isn't the enemy , they're simply someone trying to navigate their own emotional landscape.

Key Research Findings: The 58% Success Factor

Marcus had been dreading Monday morning meetings for months. As a marketing director at a growing company, he found himself constantly butting heads with colleagues who seemed to shoot down his ideas before he'd even finished presenting them. He'd started to believe that office politics were just an inevitable part of corporate life, frustrating, but unchangeable. The turning point came during a particularly tense brainstorming session. Instead of immediately defending his latest campaign concept when faced with criticism, Marcus took a breath and asked, "Help me understand your concerns. What specifically worries you about this approach?" The room's energy shifted. His colleague Monica, who had been his biggest critic, explained that she was worried about the timeline conflicting with the product launch. Another team member shared concerns about budget constraints that Marcus hadn't considered."I realized I had been taking their feedback personally," Marcus reflects. "I was so focused on proving my ideas were good that I couldn't hear what they were actually trying to tell me.

"Dr. Travis Brad berry, co-author of "Emotional Intelligence 2.0," observes that "emotional intelligence is responsible for 58% of job performance in all types of jobs." This isn't just about being nice, it's about creating environments where people can do their best work. Marcus began approaching meetings differently. Instead of coming in with fully formed proposals, he'd present initial concepts and invite collaboration. He learned to read the room , noticing when people seemed overwhelmed or disengaged, and adjusting his approach accordingly. The results were remarkable. His team began generating more creative solutions, and Marcus found himself enjoying work again. More importantly, he discovered that emotional intelligence wasn't about managing others' emotions , it was about understanding how emotions (including his own) influenced group dynamics.

Building Deeper Connections Through Empathy

Lisa had always prided herself on being logical and levelheaded. She made decisions based on facts, not feelings, and she couldn't understand why her teenage daughter Emily seemed to live in a constant state of emotional turbulence. Their relationship had become a series of explosive arguments followed by tense silences. Lisa would approach Emily's problems with practical solutions, only to be met with accusations that she "didn't understand" or "didn't care." It was exhausting and confusing. Everything changed when Lisa began paying attention to her own emotional responses during these interactions. She noticed that Emily's big feelings triggered anxiety in her , a need to fix everything quickly so she could feel in control again. Her logical advice was actually her way of managing her own discomfort with Emily's emotional intensity. "I had to learn that my discomfort with big emotions wasn't Emily's problem to solve," Lisa explains. "When I could stay calm with her feelings, she felt safer sharing what was really going on."

Dr. Susan David, author of "*Emotional Agility*," reminds us that "emotions are data, not direction." They provide information about our inner state and our needs, but they don't have to dictate our actions. When Lisa learned to observe her emotional responses without immediately acting on them, she could be more present for Emily's experience. This meant sitting with Emma's frustration about friend drama without immediately jumping to problem solving mode. It meant acknowledging Emily's disappointment about not making the soccer team without trying to minimize her feelings. Paradoxically, when Lisa stopped trying to fix Emily's emotions, their relationship began to heal. The skill Lisa developed , what psychologists call emotional awareness , is foundational to emotional intelligence. It's the ability to notice our feelings as they arise and understand what they're telling us about our needs, fears, and desires. This awareness gives us choice in how we respond.

E-Q Professional Settings: A Game-Changer for Success

David thought he was being helpful. As a senior manager at a consulting firm, he prided himself on his direct communication style and his ability to quickly identify problems. When team members brought him issues, he'd immediately launch into solutions mode, often cutting them off mid sentence to share his insights. He was genuinely surprised when his annual review included feedback that he was "difficult to approach" and "dismissive of others' ideas." From David's perspective, he was being efficient and results oriented. From his team's perspective, he was being inconsiderate and overwhelming. The wake-up call came during a team meeting when David noticed that people had stopped bringing up problems altogether. When he asked why, one brave colleague said, "We've learned that when we come to you with issues, you take over the conversation. Sometimes we just need to be heard first."

Dr. Daniel Siegel, a clinical psychiatrist and researcher, describes this phenomenon as "feeling felt", the human need to sense that another person truly understands our experience. David realized he had been so focused on solving problems that he'd forgotten to help his team feel heard. He began experimenting with what he called "listening first." When someone brought him a problem, he'd ask questions to understand their perspective before offering solutions. He learned to read nonverbal cues, noticing when someone seemed frustrated or overwhelmed, and adjusting his approach accordingly. "I discovered that most of the time, people already knew what they needed to do," David reflects. "They just needed someone to listen and validate their thinking. When I stopped trying to be the smartest person in the room and started focusing on being the most supportive, everything changed." This shift from talking to listening, from solving to understanding, transformed David's leadership style. His team began bringing him more complex problems because they trusted that he would truly hear them. Paradoxically, by focusing less on having all the answers, David became more effective at helping his team find solutions.

Mastering Self-Regulation Under Pressure

Jane's hands were shaking as she walked into the conference room. She was about to present her quarterly results to the executive team, and despite having excellent numbers to share, she felt like she might vomit. The familiar voice in her head was already running through everything that could go wrong. For years, Jane had tried to overcome her presentation anxiety by preparing more thoroughly, rehearsing until she could recite her material perfectly. But no amount of preparation seemed to quiet the storm in her stomach before big presentations. The breakthrough came when Jane stopped trying to eliminate her anxiety and started getting curious about it. What was this feeling trying to tell her? She realized that her anxiety was actually a sign that something mattered to her , that she cared about doing well and making a good impression.

Dr. Brené Brown, research professor and author of "Daring Greatly," notes that "vulnerability is not weakness; it's our greatest measure of courage." Jane learned to re-frame her nervous energy as excitement about the opportunity to share her work. She developed a pre-presentation routine that worked with her anxiety rather than against it. She'd arrive early to set up and get comfortable in the space. She'd take a few minutes to remind herself that her colleagues wanted her to succeed, not fail. Most importantly, she'd acknowledge her nervousness: "I'm feeling anxious because this matters to me, and that's okay." During presentations, when she felt her heart racing, Jane learned to slow down her speaking pace and make eye contact with friendly faces. She discovered that her anxiety often peaked in the first few minutes, then naturally subsided as she got into the flow of sharing information she knew well. "I realized that trying to be perfect was actually making me less effective," Jane explains. "When I could be authentic about being nervous, people connected with me more. They saw me as human, not just as someone delivering information." This shift from fighting emotions to working with them is central to emotional intelligence. Our feelings aren't obstacles to overcome , they're information about what matters to us and what we need. When we can listen to this information without being overwhelmed by it, we can make better decisions and show up more authentically in our relationships.

The Conflict Transformation

When business partners Jake and Rachel started their graphic design agency five years ago, they were best friends who shared a vision of creating meaningful work while maintaining work life balance. But as the company grew, so did their disagreements about direction and strategy. Jake wanted to expand aggressively, taking on bigger clients and hiring more staff. Rachel preferred to focus on their existing clients and maintain the personal touch that had made them successful. Their discussions about the future had become heated arguments, with each trying to convince the other they were wrong. The breaking point came during a particularly difficult conversation when Rachel said, "I feel like you don't value what we've built here." Jake's immediate reaction was to defend his vision, but something in Rachel's tone made him pause. "Can you help me understand what you're afraid of?" he asked instead. The question opened a door they hadn't walked through in months. Rachel shared her fear that rapid growth would compromise the quality and personal relationships that had always been their strength. Jake realized that his push for expansion was driven by his own anxiety about financial security and staying competitive. As mediation expert William Ury notes, "The single most important skill in negotiation is the ability to listen , not just to the words, but to the person behind them." When Jake and Rachel could hear each other's underlying concerns rather than just their positions, they found common ground. They discovered they both wanted financial stability and meaningful work , they just had different ideas about how to achieve those goals. This understanding led to a compromise: measured growth that would increase their security without sacrificing their values. More importantly, they learned to approach future disagreements as collaborative problem-solving rather than adversarial debates. They developed a practice of starting difficult conversations by acknowledging what they both wanted to achieve. Conflict, they realized, wasn't a sign that their partnership was failing , it was information about different perspectives and needs. When they could approach their differences with curiosity rather than defensiveness, they found solutions that served both their interests.

The Practice of Emotional Intelligence

Developing emotional intelligence isn't about achieving perfection or never feeling difficult emotions. It's about building awareness and skills that help us navigate life's complexities with greater wisdom and compassion.

Dr. Marc Brackett, director of the Yale Center for Emotional Intelligence, emphasizes that "emotions matter because they drive learning, decision-making, creativity, relationships, and health." When we can work skillfully with emotions . both our own and others' , we create better outcomes in every area of life. The journey begins with simple awareness. Throughout your day, notice what you're feeling without immediately judging it as good or bad. When you feel frustrated, get curious about what need isn't being met. When you feel anxious, ask what this feeling might be trying to protect. Practice perspective taking in your relationships. When someone's behavior puzzles or irritates you, try to imagine what they might be experiencing. Most people are doing the best they can with the resources and information available to them. In conflicts, focus on understanding before being understood. Ask questions that help you see the situation from the other person's perspective. Look for the underlying interests and needs that might be driving their position. Remember that emotional intelligence is a practice, not a destination. Some days you'll handle challenging situations with grace and wisdom. Other days you'll react in ways that surprise or disappoint you. Both are part of the human experience.

Creating Ripple Effects

The beautiful thing about developing emotional intelligence is that it creates positive ripple effects in all your relationships. When you become more emotionally aware and skilled, you model these qualities for others. Your family members, colleagues, and friends begin to feel safer being authentic around you. Children especially benefit from being around emotionally intelligent adults. When they see us managing our emotions skillfully and responding to theirs with understanding, they learn that feelings are manageable and that relationships can be safe spaces for authentic expression. As you continue developing these skills, you'll likely find that relationships become more satisfying, conflicts become opportunities for deeper understanding, and daily interactions become more pleasant. You'll feel more confident in your ability to handle whatever emotional challenges arise. The investment in emotional intelligence pays dividends in every area of life. It's not just about feeling better , though that's certainly a benefit. It's about creating a life where you can show up as your best self in your relationships and work, where you can navigate challenges with resilience, and where you can contribute to creating more understanding and connection in the world. The path forward is not about becoming someone different, but about becoming more fully yourself, aware, skilled, and compassionate in your dealings with the rich emotional landscape of human experience.

Chapter 9: Coping with Loneliness: Finding Connection in a Disconnected World

Amanda stared at her phone screen, scrolling through endless social media feeds filled with friends' vacation photos and celebration posts. Despite being surrounded by hundreds of online connections, she felt more alone than ever. At 28, successful in her career and living in a vibrant city, she couldn't shake the persistent ache of isolation that had become her constant companion. Amanda's story reflects a growing reality for millions of people worldwide, we're living through an unprecedented epidemic of loneliness.

The Hidden Epidemic

In our hyper connected digital age, loneliness has emerged as one of the most pressing public health challenges of our time. Our latest brief report is based on a nationally representative survey of adults conducted in May 2024 and suggests 21% of adults in the U. S. feel lonely, while 30% of adults say they have experienced feelings of loneliness at least once a week over the past year. These statistics tell only part of the story. About 1 in 3 adults in the U. S. report feeling lonely, and approximately 20% of U. S. adults are experiencing daily loneliness, as indicated by a recent Gallup survey. The scope of this crisis extends far beyond mere numbers.

The Loneliness Epidemic: Research led by Dr. Steven Cole at UCLA reveals that chronic loneliness doesn't just impact our emotional well-being, it fundamentally alters our biology at the genetic level. In a groundbreaking 2007 study published in Genome Biology, Cole and his colleagues identified 209 genes that were differentially expressed in the immune cells of chronically lonely individuals compared to socially connected people. The findings show that feelings of social isolation are linked to alterations in the activity of genes that drive inflammation, the first response of the immune system. Specifically, genes that activate immune system inflammation were over expressed, while those that regulate antibody production and antiviral responses were under expressed. This altered immune response makes lonely people markedly more vulnerable to outside threats such as viruses and bacteria, while also putting them under attack from within by their own bodies. Further research by Dr. Cole's team found that both lonely humans and monkeys had higher levels of inflammatory white blood cells in their blood due to increased production of immature immune cells (Cole et al., 2007).

Understanding the Roots of Modern Loneliness

The causes of our loneliness epidemic are complex and multifaceted. We live in an era of unprecedented connectivity, yet genuine connection seems increasingly elusive. Several factors contribute to this paradox:

The Digital Paradox While technology promised to bring us closer together, it has often created barriers to authentic connection. Social media platforms, designed to foster interaction, frequently leave users feeling more isolated and inadequate. The curated nature of online personas creates unrealistic comparisons and diminishes the quality of genuine relationships.

Social Fragmentation: Traditional community structures that once provided natural opportunities for connection, extended families, religious congregations, neighborhood networks, have weakened or disappeared entirely. Many people now live in environments where they barely know their neighbors, let alone maintain meaningful relationships with them.

The Mobility Culture: Modern society's emphasis on career mobility means people frequently relocate, leaving behind established social networks. The effort required to rebuild these connections in new environments can be overwhelming, leading many to remain socially isolated.

Changing Work Patterns: The rise of remote work, while offering flexibility, has eliminated many informal social interactions that occur in traditional office settings. The casual conversations, shared meals, and spontaneous collaborations that build workplace relationships have largely disappeared.

The Psychological Architecture of Loneliness

To effectively address loneliness, we must first understand its psychological underpinnings. Loneliness is not simply being alone, it's the subjective experience of feeling disconnected from others, regardless of the actual number of social contacts a person has.

Dr. John Cacioppo, a pioneering researcher in loneliness studies, identified loneliness as an evolved signal, much like hunger or thirst, that motivates us to seek social connection essential for survival. However, in our modern context, this signal can become chronically activated, leading to a cycle of negative thinking and social withdrawal. The research reveals fascinating patterns in how loneliness affects different age groups. Loneliness peaked in the late 20s, mid-50s, and late 80s, suggesting that life transitions, whether entering adulthood, facing midlife challenges, or dealing with aging, create particular vulnerability to social isolation.

Michael's Midlife Crisis

Michael, a 52 year old marketing executive, found himself increasingly isolated after his divorce. His children lived with their mother, his social circle had revolved around couples' activities, and his demanding work schedule left little time for building new relationships. Despite having colleagues and acquaintances, Michael felt profoundly alone. His story illustrates how major life transitions can trigger periods of intense loneliness, particularly when existing social structures are disrupted.

The Ripple Effects: How Loneliness Impacts Mental Health

The relationship between loneliness and mental health is both profound and bidirectional. In the report, 81% of adults who were lonely also said they suffered with anxiety or depression compared to 29% of those who were less lonely. This statistic reveals the intricate web connecting social isolation and psychological distress. Loneliness doesn't just contribute to mental health problems, it fundamentally alters how we perceive and interact with the world. Chronic loneliness can lead to:

Cognitive Distortions: Lonely individuals often develop negative thought patterns, interpreting neutral social interactions as rejections or signs of disinterest. This creates a self-fulfilling prophecy where anticipation of rejection leads to withdrawal, which in turn reinforces the original belief.

Hyper-vigilance: The lonely brain becomes hypersensitive to social threats, constantly scanning for signs of exclusion or rejection. This heightened state of alertness is exhausting and prevents the relaxation necessary for genuine connection.

Emotional Dysregulation: Loneliness disrupts the brain's ability to regulate emotions effectively, leading to increased reactivity, difficulty managing stress, and reduced capacity for empathy.

Breaking the Cycle: Evidence Based Interventions

The good news is that loneliness is treatable, and research has identified several effective intervention strategies. Psychological treatment, social support interventions, and social and emotional skills training appeared to be the most effective intervention strategies in reducing loneliness. Meta analyses of loneliness interventions have identified four primary approaches: improving social skills, enhancing social support, increasing opportunities for social contact, and addressing maladaptive social cognition. Each approach addresses different aspects of the loneliness experience.

1. Cognitive Restructuring: Changing the Inner Dialogue

The most effective interventions often begin with addressing the distorted thinking patterns that perpetuate loneliness. Cognitive behavioral therapy (CBT) techniques help individuals identify and challenge negative assumptions about social interactions.

Practical Exercise: The "Social Evidence Log"

Keep a daily record of social interactions, noting:

»What happened (objective facts)

»Your initial interpretation

»Alternative explanations

»Evidence for and against your interpretation

»A more balanced perspective

This practice helps break the cycle of negative interpretation that keeps lonely individuals trapped in isolation.

2.Social Skills Development: Building Connection Competencies

Many people struggling with loneliness lack the social skills necessary for initiating and maintaining relationships. This isn't a character flaw, it's a learnable set of competencies.

Key social skills for connection include:

Active Listening: Moving beyond waiting for your turn to speak, active listening involves fully engaging with others' words, emotions, and underlying meanings. Practice reflecting back what you hear, asking clarifying questions, and showing genuine interest in others' experiences.

Emotional Intelligence: Developing the ability to recognize, understand, and respond appropriately to your own emotions and those of others. This includes learning to express vulnerability appropriately and offer support to others.

Conversation Skills: Learning to initiate conversations, maintain dialogue, and gracefully end interactions. This includes mastering the art of small talk as a pathway to deeper connection.

Conflict Resolution: Developing skills to navigate disagreements and tensions in relationships without permanent damage to the connection.

3. *Social Support Enhancement:* Building Your Network

Creating a robust social support system requires intentional effort and strategic thinking. Research shows that quality matters more than quantity, a few deep, meaningful relationships are far more valuable than numerous superficial connections.

Mapping Your Social Network:

Create a visual map of your current relationships, categorizing them by:

»Immediate family and close friends

»Workplace relationships

»Community connections

»Acquaintances with potential for deeper connection

»Professional or interest based networks

Identify gaps and opportunities for strengthening existing relationships or developing new ones.

The 3-3-3 Rules

Aim to have three different types of social connection:

- *3 Close Intimates:* People with whom you can share your deepest thoughts and feelings
- *3 Regular Companions:* Friends you see regularly for activities and casual conversation
- 3 *Broader Networks:* Groups or communities that provide a sense of belonging and shared purpose

4.Increasing Social Opportunities: Creating Pathways to Connection

Loneliness often persists because individuals lack opportunities for meaningful social interaction. This is particularly challenging for those who work from home, have moved to new areas, or have experienced major life transitions.

Strategies for expanding social opportunities:

Structured Activities: Join clubs, classes, or groups centered around shared interests. The structure provides natural conversation starters and reduces the pressure of initiating interaction.

Volunteering: Helping others creates natural opportunities for connection while providing a sense of purpose and meaning. Research shows that volunteering can significantly reduce feelings of loneliness.

Regular Commitments: Establish recurring social commitments, weekly coffee with a friend, monthly book club, or regular workout partner. Consistency builds deeper relationships over time.

Proximity Advantage: Prioritize connections with people you see regularly, neighbors, colleagues, or fellow commuters. Frequent, low pressure interactions often evolve into meaningful relationships.

Susan's Community Connection

Susan, a 45 year-old teacher who had recently moved to a new city, felt overwhelmed by the prospect of building new friendships. She started small by joining a local hiking group that met every Saturday morning. Initially, she barely spoke to anyone, but the shared activity provided natural conversation starters. Over several months, she began grabbing coffee with other hikers after their walks. These casual interactions gradually deepened into genuine friendships. A year later, Susan had built a solid social network and felt truly connected to her new community.

The Role of Technology: Tool or Barrier?

Technology's impact on loneliness is nuanced and depends largely on how it's used. While social media can contribute to isolation, digital tools can also facilitate meaningful connection when used intentionally.

Helpful technology practices:

Video Calls Over Text: Prioritize face to face interaction, even when digital. Video calls provide visual and emotional cues that text based communication lacks.

Online Communities: Join online groups centered around specific interests or challenges. These communities can provide support and connection, particularly for those with niche interests or circumstances.

Digital Detox: Regular breaks from social media can help reset your relationship with technology and create space for in person interactions.

Connection Apps: Apps designed specifically for making friends or finding activity partners can be valuable tools for expanding social networks.

Research on technology enabled mental health support interventions show that virtual one on one support, group support, and self guided resources can increase feelings of connection. The key is using technology as a bridge to human connection rather than a replacement for it.

The Kindness Connection

Research has revealed an unexpected pathway to reducing loneliness: acts of kindness toward others. Promoting the provision of social support through small acts of kindness to neighbors has the potential to reduce loneliness, social isolation and social anxiety, and promote neighbor hood relationships.

When we focus on helping others, several beneficial things happen:

»We shift attention away from our own distress

»We experience a sense of purpose and meaning

»We create opportunities for positive social interaction

»We build our social identity as helpful and caring individuals

The Kindness Challenge: Commit to performing one small act of kindness each day for a week. This could be as simple as holding a door, complimenting a stranger, or checking in on a neighbor. Notice how these interactions affect your mood and sense of connection.

Building Emotional Resilience

Developing resilience to loneliness involves building internal resources that help you cope with inevitable periods of isolation. Life circumstances will sometimes separate us from others, but resilient individuals can maintain their emotional well-being during these times.

Resilience building strategies:

Self-Compassion: Treat yourself with the same kindness you would offer a good friend. Loneliness often involves harsh self-criticism that amplifies distress.

Meaning-Making: Develop a sense of purpose that transcends immediate social connections. This might involve creative pursuits, spiritual practices, or contributing to causes larger than yourself.

Solitude Skills: Learn to enjoy your own company through activities like reading, walking in nature, or pursuing hobbies that bring you joy.

Physical Health: Regular exercise, adequate sleep, and good nutrition support emotional resilience and provide natural opportunities for social interaction.

The Workplace Connection

Given that many adults spend the majority of their waking hours at work, workplace relationships play a crucial role in combating loneliness. The shift to remote work has highlighted the importance of intentional connection in professional settings.

Strategies for workplace connection:

Coffee Conversations: Schedule regular informal check-ins with colleagues, focusing on personal interests and experiences beyond work tasks.

Mentorship: Both mentoring others and seeking mentorship create meaningful professional relationships that often extend beyond work.

Team Building: Participate in or organize team activities that allow colleagues to connect as individuals rather than just professional roles.

Collaboration: Seek opportunities to work closely with others on projects, which naturally builds stronger relationships.

Community Solutions: Beyond Individual Action

While individual strategies are essential, addressing the loneliness epidemic requires community level interventions. Communities that prioritize social connection create environments where loneliness is less likely to develop and persist.

Community based approaches include:

Social Prescribing: Healthcare providers can "prescribe" social activities, support groups, or community programs as part of treatment for loneliness and related mental health issues.

Public Space Design: Creating spaces that encourage social interaction, community gardens, public squares, neighborhood centers ,provides natural opportunities for connection.

Inter-generational Programs: Initiatives that bring together people of different ages combat loneliness while fostering mutual understanding and support.

Neighborhood Networks: Organized efforts to strengthen local connections through block parties, skill sharing programs, or mutual aid networks.

When to Seek Professional Help

While many people can address loneliness through self-help strategies and community connections, professional support may be necessary when:

»Loneliness persists despite consistent efforts to build connections

»Feelings of isolation are accompanied by depression, anxiety, or other mental health symptoms

»Loneliness is interfering with daily functioning or quality of life

»You're experiencing thoughts of self-harm or suicide

Mental health professionals can provide specialized interventions, including:

Cognitive behavioral therapy specifically designed for loneliness

Group therapy focused on social skills and connection

Treatment for underlying mental health conditions that may contribute to isolation

Medication when appropriate for related depression or anxiety

The Path Forward: A Connected Future

As we move forward in an increasingly complex world, the need for genuine human connection becomes ever more critical. The loneliness epidemic is not an inevitable consequence of modern life, it's a challenge we can address through intentional individual actions and collective community efforts. The journey from loneliness to connection is rarely linear. It involves setbacks, small victories, and gradual progress. The key is persistence, self compassion, and the willingness to be vulnerable with others. Every small step toward connection, whether it's a smile to a stranger, a text to an old friend, or joining a new group, contributes to both individual healing and community resilience. Remember that seeking connection is not a sign of weakness but a fundamental human need. In a world that often prioritizes individual achievement over communal well-being, choosing to prioritize relationships is both a personal act of self-care and a radical act of hope for our collective future. The epidemic of loneliness is real, but so is our capacity for connection. By understanding the roots of isolation, developing practical skills for building relationships, and creating communities that support social connection, we can begin to heal not just our individual loneliness but the broader social fabric that binds us together. In the end, the antidote to loneliness isn't just finding people to be with, it's discovering how to be fully present with others and allowing them to be present with us.

Action Steps for Connection

1. *Start with self assessment:* Use the loneliness assessment tools available through mental health resources to understand your current level of social connection.

2. *Identify your connection style:* Reflect on what types of social interactions energize you and which ones feel draining. Build on your natural strengths while gradually expanding your comfort zone.

3. *Create a connection plan:* Set specific, measurable goals for building relationships. This might include reaching out to one person each week, joining a new group, or scheduling regular social activities.

4. *Practice daily micro-connections:* Engage in small social interactions throughout your day, chat with a cashier, compliment a colleague, or wave to a neighbor.

5. *Embrace vulnerability:* Share something meaningful about yourself with someone you trust. Vulnerability is the pathway to deeper connection.

6. *Be patient with the process:* Building meaningful relationships takes time. Focus on consistency rather than in-tensity, and celebrate small progress along the way.

The journey from loneliness to connection is one of the most important paths we can travel. It requires courage, patience, and the willingness to risk rejection in pursuit of authentic human connection. But the rewards, improved mental health, greater life satisfaction, and a sense of belonging, make every effort worthwhile. In a world that often feels disconnected, choosing to connect is both a personal victory and a gift to everyone whose life you to touch.

Chapter 10: Seeking Help Breaking the Stigma Around Mental Health

The text message sat on Esther's phone for three hours before she finally hit send: "I think I need help." Those five words represented weeks of internal struggle, sleepless nights, and the weight of carrying a burden she could no longer bear alone. As a successful marketing executive, Esther had always prided herself on being strong, capable, and in control. But anxiety had crept into her life like a thief in the night, stealing her confidence and leaving her feeling like a stranger in her own skin. Esther's hesitation wasn't unusual. Despite living in an era of unprecedented mental health awareness, the stigma surrounding seeking help remains a formidable barrier. The fear of being judged, labeled, or seen as weak continues to prevent millions from accessing the support they desperately need.

The Silent Epidemic

Mental health challenges are far more common than most people realize. 1 in 5 U. S. adults experience mental illness each year, yet the conversation around mental health often happens in whispers, shrouded in shame and misunderstanding. This silence comes at a devastating cost, not just to individuals, but to families, communities, and society as a whole. The statistics paint a sobering picture of how stigma operates in our daily lives. A 2022 national poll from the American Psychiatric Association (A-P-A) found that mental health stigma is still a major challenge in the workplace. About half (48%) of workers say they can discuss mental health openly and honestly with their supervisor, down from 56% in 2021 and 62% in 2020. This downward trend suggests that despite increased awareness, the barriers to seeking help may actually be growing stronger.

Dr. Sarah Chen, a leading psychiatrist at Johns Hopkins University, explains the paradox: "We've made tremendous progress in understanding mental health from a clinical perspective, but culturally, we're still fighting the same battles. People know more about depression and anxiety than ever before, yet they're increasingly afraid to admit they're struggling."

The Many Faces of Stigma

Stigma doesn't exist in a vacuum, it manifests in multiple forms, each creating its own barriers to healing and recovery.

Public Stigma: The Weight of Others' Judgment

Public stigma refers to the negative attitudes, beliefs, and behaviors that society holds toward people with mental health conditions. It's the raised eyebrows when someone mentions therapy, the hushed conversations about a colleague's "breakdown," or the assumption that mental illness equals weakness or instability.

Consider the story of Michael, a 28 year old teacher who experienced his first panic attack during a parent-teacher conference. Word spread quickly through the small school community, and suddenly, parents were questioning his ability to handle their children's education. "I went from being a respected educator to someone people whispered about in the hallways," Michael recalls. "The stigma was almost harder to deal with than the panic attacks themselves."

Self-Stigma: The Internal Battle

Perhaps even more damaging than public stigma is self stigma, the internalization of negative beliefs about mental health. When individuals accept and apply stigmatizing attitudes to themselves, it creates a vicious cycle of shame and avoidance.

Dr. Patrick Corrigan, a renowned researcher in mental health stigma, notes, "Self-stigma is particularly insidious because it attacks from within. People begin to believe they're fundamentally flawed or that their struggles are a personal failing rather than a medical condition."

Lisa, a 45-year-old accountant, battled depression for years before seeking help. "I kept telling myself that I should be able to handle this on my own," she explains. "I was convinced that needing help meant I was weak, that I was somehow less than other people who seemed to have it all together."

Structural Stigma: Systems That Fail

Structural stigma operates at an institutional level, embedded in policies, practices, and systems that systematically discriminate against people with mental health conditions. This might include insurance companies that provide inadequate coverage for mental health services, employers who don't offer mental health benefits, or healthcare systems that treat mental health as secondary to physical health. The impact of structural stigma is particularly evident in workplace policies. A recent study found that while 83% of employees report work related stress, only 40% feel comfortable discussing mental health concerns with their employers. This disconnect highlights how organizational cultures can inadvertently perpetuate stigma through silence and inaction.

The Ripple Effect: How Stigma Spreads

Stigma doesn't remain confined to the individual experiencing it, it spreads through families, communities, and entire cultures, creating widespread barriers to mental health care.

Family Dynamics

Mental health stigma often begins at home. Families may struggle with their own understanding of mental health, leading to responses that, while well intentioned, can be harmful. Comments like "just think positive thoughts" or "you have nothing to be depressed about" minimize the person's experience and can increase feelings of isolation.

Maria, a college student who struggled with anxiety, describes her family's reaction: "My parents kept saying I was just stressed about school and that I needed to pray more. They meant well, but their inability to understand what I was going through made me feel even more alone."

Cultural Considerations

Mental health stigma varies significantly across cultures. In many Asian cultures, for example, mental health issues are often viewed as bringing shame to the entire family. This cultural context can make seeking help feel like a betrayal of family honor.

Dr. Amy Nguyen, a cultural psychiatrist, explains: "In collectivist cultures, the individual's mental health is often seen as a reflection of the family's success or failure. This creates additional pressure to hide struggles and avoid seeking help." Similarly, in many Latino communities, the concept of "personalismo", the importance of personal relationships and family loyalty, can make it difficult for individuals to seek outside help for mental health concerns.

The Science of Stigma: What Research Reveals

Recent research has provided valuable insights into how stigma operates and its impact on mental health outcomes.

The Neurobiological Impact

Studies using brain imaging technology have shown that experiencing stigma activates the same neural pathways as physical pain. This research, led by Dr. Naomi Eisenberger at UCLA, demonstrates that social rejection and stigma create genuine neurological distress, not just emotional discomfort.

"When we say that stigma 'hurts,' we're not speaking metaphorically," Dr. Eisenberger explains. "The brain processes social rejection using the same systems it uses to process physical pain. This is why stigma can be so debilitating and why it has such a profound impact on mental health."

The Delay Effect

Research consistently shows that stigma leads to significant delays in seeking mental health treatment. On average, people wait nearly a decade between the onset of symptoms and their first contact with a mental health professional. This delay can have serious consequences, as early intervention is crucial for effective treatment.

Dr. Ronald Kessler, a psychiatric epidemiologist at Harvard Medical School, notes: "The longer someone waits to seek help, the more entrenched their condition becomes. What might have been easily treatable in the early stages can become a chronic, life altering condition."

The Recovery Paradox

Interestingly, research has shown that people who experience less stigma have better treatment outcomes, regardless of the severity of their initial symptoms. This suggests that stigma itself can be a significant barrier to recovery, independent of the underlying mental health condition.

Breaking Through: Stories of Courage

Despite the challenges, countless individuals have found the courage to seek help and break through the barriers of stigma. Their stories offer hope and practical insights for others facing similar struggles.

The Executive's Journey

Thomas, a 52 year old CEO, experienced severe depression following a series of professional setbacks. For months, he struggled in silence, convinced that seeking help would damage his reputation and career prospects. "I was terrified that if word got out, I'd be seen as unstable or unfit to lead," Thomas recalls. "But the depression was consuming me. I was making poor decisions, my relationships were suffering, and I was becoming someone I didn't recognize." The turning point came when Thomas's wife staged an intervention, bringing together several close friends and family members. "They didn't judge me or tell me to 'snap out of it,'" he explains. "They simply said they were worried and wanted to help." Thomas began seeing a therapist and eventually started taking medication. Six months later, he made a difficult decision: he shared his mental health journey with his company's leadership team and, eventually, with all employees during a company wide meeting. "The response was overwhelming," Thomas says. "Dozens of employees reached out to share their own struggles. We ended up completely revamping our mental health benefits and creating a culture where seeking help is seen as a sign of strength, not weakness."

The Student's Awakening

Ashley, a 20 year old college student, struggled with eating disorders and anxiety throughout high school. Despite her symptoms, she managed to maintain excellent grades and participate in numerous extracurricular activities, leading everyone to assume she was thriving. "I was the perfect student on the outside," Ashley explains, "but inside, I was falling apart. I thought seeking help would mean admitting I was a fraud." The catalyst for change came during her freshman year of college when a friend noticed her skipping meals and confronted her with compassion rather than judgment. "She didn't try to fix me or give me advice," Ashley recalls. "She just said, 'I'm worried about you, and I think you deserve to feel better.'" Ashley began seeing a counselor at the student health center and joined a support group for students with eating disorders. "I discovered that I wasn't alone," she says. "There were other high achieving students who were struggling too. It helped me realize that needing help doesn't make you weak, it makes you human."

The Celebrity Effect: High Profile Advocacy

The involvement of celebrities in mental health advocacy has played a significant role in reducing stigma and encouraging people to seek help. When public figures share their own struggles, it can have a powerful normalizing effect.

Lady Gaga is perhaps one of the more recognized celebrity mental health advocates, particularly since she started the Born This Way Foundation to help those struggling with mental illness. Her openness about her own experiences with anxiety and depression has helped countless fans feel less alone in their struggles.

Demi Lovato, a longtime mental health advocate, has bravely shared her journey with the public. She has spoken about her experience with bipolar disorder, addiction, and bulimia. Demi's openness has helped dispel stereotypes and fostered honest discussions about mental health.

Dr. Jennifer Aaker, a social psychologist at Stanford University, has studied the impact of celebrity disclosure on mental health stigma. "When celebrities share their struggles, it creates what we call 'parasocial contact,'" she explains. "People feel connected to these public figures, and their disclosure can challenge stereotypes and reduce stigma on a large scale."

The Workplace Revolution

One of the most significant battlegrounds for mental health stigma is the workplace. Progressive companies are beginning to recognize that mental health isn't just a personal issue, it's a business imperative.

Leading by Example

Microsoft has emerged as a leader in workplace mental health advocacy. The company provides comprehensive mental health benefits, including therapy and counseling services, and has trained managers to recognize signs of mental health struggles in their team members.

Satya Nadella, Microsoft's CEO, has spoken publicly about the importance of mental health in the workplace: "We have a responsibility to create an environment where people feel safe to be vulnerable, to ask for help, and to prioritize their mental well-being."

The Ripple Effect

Companies that prioritize mental health often see positive outcomes beyond employee well being. A study by the World Health Organization found that for every dollar invested in mental health treatment, there's a four dollar return in improved health and productivity.

Jennifer, a human resources director at a Fortune 500 company, describes the transformation she's witnessed: "When we started talking openly about mental health and providing resources, we saw a dramatic decrease in absenteeism and turnover. Employees became more engaged, more creative, and more collaborative."

The Technology Revolution

Digital platforms and mental health apps are playing an increasingly important role in reducing barriers to care and normalizing conversations about mental health.

Accessible Entry Points

Apps like Head space, Calm, and Better Help have made mental health resources more accessible than ever before. These platforms allow people to explore mental health support without the fear of judgment that might come with traditional therapy.

Dr. John Torous, a digital psychiatry expert at Harvard Medical School, notes: "Digital platforms can serve as a bridge for people who are hesitant to seek traditional therapy. They provide a low pressure way to explore mental health resources and can help normalize the idea of seeking help."

The Community Effect

Online support groups and forums have created communities where people can share their experiences and find support from others who understand their struggles. These digital spaces can be particularly valuable for individuals who feel isolated in their offline communities.

Sarah, a 34 year old mother who struggled with postpartum depression, found support through an online community: "I felt like I was the only one who wasn't blissfully happy after having a baby. Finding other women who understood what I was going through probably saved my life."

Professional Perspectives: What Experts Know

Mental health professionals have unique insights into the impact of stigma and the most effective strategies for overcoming it.

The Therapeutic Relationship

Dr. Marsha Linehan, creator of Dialectical Behavior Therapy (D B T), emphasizes the importance of the therapeutic relationship in overcoming stigma: "The first thing we need to do is create a space where people feel genuinely accepted and understood. When clients feel judged, they shut down. When they feel accepted, they open up."

The Power of Validation

Validation, the practice of acknowledging and accepting someone's experience without judgment, is crucial for overcoming self stigma. Dr. Daniel Siegel, a clinical professor of psychiatry at UCLA, explains: "When we feel truly seen and understood, it activates neural pathways associated with safety and connection. This is the foundation for healing."

Integrated Care Models

Many mental health professionals advocate for integrated care models that treat mental health alongside physical health. This approach can help reduce the artificial separation between mental and physical health that contributes to stigma.

Dr. Susan McQuaid, a family physician who specializes in integrated care, notes: "When we treat mental health as just another aspect of overall health, it becomes less stigmatized. Patients are more likely to seek help when they don't feel like they're being referred to a 'special' or 'different' kind of doctor."

Personal Strategies

1. Education and Awareness

Understanding mental health conditions from a scientific perspective can help reduce self-stigma. Learning about the biological, psychological, and social factors that contribute to mental health challenges can help individuals view their struggles as medical conditions rather than personal failings.

2. Language Matters

The way we talk about mental health influences how we think about it. Using person first language ("person with depression" rather than "depressed person") and avoiding stigmatizing terms can help reduce both self-stigma and public stigma.

3. Finding Your Tribe

Connecting with others who have similar experiences can provide validation and support. This might involve joining support groups, online communities, or simply opening up to trusted friends and family members.

4. Gradual Disclosure

Sharing your mental health journey doesn't have to be an all-or-nothing proposition. Start with trusted individuals and gradually expand your circle of support as you feel more comfortable.

Community Strategies

1. Storytelling

Personal stories have the power to change hearts and minds. When people share their mental health journeys, it helps others realize they're not alone and challenges stereotypes about mental illness.

2. Education Program

Schools, workplaces, and community organizations can implement mental health education programs that provide accurate information and challenge misconceptions.

3. Contact Based Interventions

Research shows that direct contact with people who have mental health conditions is one of the most effective ways to reduce stigma. Programs that facilitate meaningful interactions between people with and without mental health conditions can be particularly powerful.

4. Media Advocacy

Encouraging responsible media coverage of mental health issues can help reduce stigma. This includes promoting accurate portrayals of mental illness and avoiding sensationalized or stigmatizing language.

The Role of Healthcare Systems

Healthcare systems play a crucial role in either perpetuating or reducing mental health stigma.

Training and Education

Healthcare providers need training to recognize and address their own biases about mental health. This includes understanding how stigma affects patient care and learning to provide compassionate, nonjudgmental treatment.

Dr. Arthur Kleinmann, a medical anthropologist at Harvard Medical School, emphasizes: "Healthcare providers are not immune to the cultural biases that surround mental health. We need to actively work to identify and address these biases if we want to provide effective care."

Integrated Care Models

Healthcare systems that integrate mental health services with primary care can help reduce stigma by treating mental health as a routine part of overall health care.

Policy Changes

Healthcare systems can implement policies that reduce barriers to mental health care, such as improving insurance coverage, reducing wait times, and ensuring that mental health services are available in all communities.

The Path Forward: A Collective Responsibility

Breaking the stigma around mental health isn't the responsibility of any single group, it requires collective action from individuals, families, communities, healthcare systems, and society as a whole.

Individual Actions

Every person can play a role in reducing mental health stigma:

»*Educate yourself* about mental health conditions and their treatments

»*Listen without judgmen*t when someone shares their mental health struggles

»*Share your own story* when you feel comfortable doing so

»*Use respectful language* when discussing mental health

»*Support mental health* initiatives in your community and workplace

»*Challenge stereotypes and misconceptions* when you encounter them

Systemic Changes

Larger systemic changes are also needed:

»*Improved mental health education* in schools and workplaces

»*Better insurance coverage* for mental health services

»*Increased funding* for mental health research and treatment

Policy changes that protect people with mental health conditions from discrimination *Cultural shifts* that normalize seeking help for mental health concerns

The Ripple Effect of Change

When individuals break through the stigma and seek help, the impact extends far beyond their own lives. Their courage to seek treatment can inspire others to do the same, creating a ripple effect of positive change.

Consider the story of a high school teacher named Robert who struggled with depression for years before seeking help. When he finally began therapy and started taking medication, his improved mental health transformed not only his own life but also his ability to connect with and support his students. "I became a better teacher because I became a better person," Robert reflects. "Students started coming to me with their own struggles, and I was able to help them in ways I never could before. Breaking through my own stigma didn't just help me, it helped dozens of young people who needed to know that it's okay to ask for help."

Hope for the Future

Despite the challenges, there are reasons for optimism. Mental health awareness is growing, particularly among younger generations who are more likely to seek help and talk openly about their mental health struggles.

The WHO MOSAIC toolkit to end stigma and discrimination in mental health provides practical, step by step guidance on how to set up anti-stigma initiatives based on principles of social contact, co-leadership by people with lived experience and meaningful collaboration. This represents a significant step forward in providing concrete tools for reducing stigma. Social media, despite its potential negative impacts, has also created new opportunities for mental health advocacy and connection. Platforms like Instagram, Tik-Tok, and Twitter are full of mental health advocates sharing their stories, providing resources, and creating communities of support.

Conclusion: The Courage to Seek Help

Esther's story, the marketing executive who struggled to send that first text asking for help, has a positive ending. Six months after beginning therapy, she describes feeling like she's gotten her life back. More importantly, she's become an advocate for mental health awareness in her workplace and community. "I used to think that seeking help was a sign of weakness," Esther reflects. "Now I realize it was one of the most courageous things I've ever done. It took strength to admit I was struggling, to reach out for help, and to do the hard work of recovery." The journey from stigma to support isn't always easy, but it's always worthwhile. Every person who breaks through the barriers of stigma and seeks help makes it a little easier for the next person to do the same. Every conversation about mental health, every act of compassion, and every story shared contributes to a cultural shift that will ultimately benefit everyone.

Mental health is not a luxury, it's a necessity. In a world that often feels overwhelming and isolating, seeking help isn't just an individual act of self care; it's a revolutionary act of hope. It's a declaration that every person deserves to live a life free from the burden of unnecessary suffering, and that healing is always possible.

The stigma around mental health has kept too many people suffering in silence for too long. But change is possible, and it starts with each of us having the courage to speak up, seek help, and support others on their journey to wellness. The conversation is changing, the barriers are falling, and help is available.

The question isn't whether you deserve help you do. The question is whether you're ready to take that first brave step toward healing. Your future self is waiting, and the world needs you at your best.

Chapter 11: The Gratitude Revolution Rewiring Your Brain for Resilience

"Gratitude is not the greatest of virtues, but the parent of all others." Cicero

The Unexpected Power of a Simple "Thank You"

Grace stared at her laptop screen, the rejection email blurring through her tears. The third job rejection in two weeks. As a single mother of two, the mounting bills felt suffocating. That evening, her seven year old daughter Mia handed her a crayon drawing, a stick figure family under a rainbow with the words "Thank you for being the best mom." In that moment, something shifted. Grace realized she'd been so focused on what was going wrong that she'd forgotten what was going right. This simple recognition became the catalyst for a profound transformation that would reshape not just her mindset, but her entire life trajectory.

This isn't just another feel good story about positive thinking. It's about a scientifically backed revolution that's quietly transforming how we understand human resilience, happiness, and success. Welcome to the gratitude revolution, where the simple act of appreciation becomes a powerful tool for rewiring your brain and transforming your life.

The Neuroscience Behind the Magic

Dr. Alex Korb, a neuroscientist at UCLA, puts it simply: "Gratitude literally changes your brain." When we practice gratitude, our brains undergo measurable changes that enhance our capacity for joy, resilience, and overall well-being.

Recent neuroimaging studies reveal that gratitude activates the brain's reward system, releasing dopamine and serotonin, the same chemicals targeted by antidepressants. More remarkably, regular gratitude practice strengthens neural pathways associated with optimism and emotional regulation while weakening those linked to anxiety and depression.

The Numbers Don't Lie

»A landmark study of 3,000 participants showed that those who wrote gratitude letters experienced a 19% increase in life satisfaction

»Brain scans revealed increased activity in the hypothalamus (which regulates stress) and ventral tegmental area (part of the brain's reward system)

»Participants showed improved sleep quality within just two weeks of starting gratitude practices

Dr. Robert Emmons, often called the "father of gratitude research," explains: "Gratitude is the ultimate performance enhancer. It doesn't just make you feel better, it makes you perform better in every area of life."

But here's what makes this truly revolutionary: these changes aren't temporary. Neuroplasticity research shows that consistent gratitude practice creates lasting structural changes in the brain, building what researchers call "gratitude neural networks."

When Life Hits Hard: Real Stories of Transformation

Mary's Miracle in the ICU

Mary Rodriguez never imagined that her darkest professional moment would become her greatest teacher. As a front line nurse during the pandemic, she watched colleagues burn out, patients struggle, and families grieve. The emotional toll was crushing. "I was drowning," Mary recalls. "Every day felt like a battle I was losing." Her turning point came during a particularly difficult shift. After losing a patient she'd grown close to, Mary found herself crying in a supply closet. Her mentor, an older nurse named Patricia, found her there. "Patricia didn't offer platitudes," Mary remembers. "She said something that changed everything: 'Find three things right now that you're grateful for. Not big things; tiny things.'" In that sterile supply closet, Mary found herself grateful for the softness of the tissues, the quiet moment away from chaos, and Patricia's presence. It seemed almost ridiculous, but something loosened in her chest. Mary began what she calls her "micro gratitude practice"; finding three tiny things to appreciate during each shift. The warmth of her coffee. A colleague's smile. A patient's improvement, however small. "It didn't change the pandemic," Mary explains. "But it changed how I moved through it. Instead of being crushed by the weight of everything wrong, I began to notice the thread of things that were right." Six months later, Mary reported significantly lower burnout scores and had become a mentor to other struggling healthcare workers. Her supervisor noted her remarkable resilience and promoted her to charge nurse.

Peter 's Business Breakthrough

Peter Kim's tech startup was hemorrhaging money. Three years of 80-hour weeks, and he was facing bankruptcy. His marriage was strained, his health was failing, and investors were pulling out. "I was bitter," Peter admits. "I felt like the world owed me success because I'd worked so hard." His therapist suggested something that initially annoyed him: a daily gratitude practice. "I thought it was touchy feely nonsense," Peter says. "But I was desperate." He started small, grateful for his morning coffee, his wife's support, his team's dedication. Gradually, the practice shifted his perspective. Instead of fixating on what investors weren't doing, he began appreciating the ones who believed in him. Instead of resenting his long hours, he felt grateful for meaningful work. "The breakthrough came when I realized that gratitude wasn't about accepting failure; it was about seeing opportunities I'd been blind to," Peter explains.

This shift in perspective led him to approach a former mentor he'd been too proud to contact. That conversation resulted in a partnership that saved his company. Today, Peter's business is thriving, and he credits his gratitude practice with saving not just his company, but his marriage and health.

Amara's Healing Journey

Amara Johnson's world shattered when she was diagnosed with breast cancer at 34. A vibrant teacher and mother of two young children, she felt her future disappearing. "The fear was consuming me," Amara reflects. "I couldn't see past the cancer to any kind of future." The initial weeks after diagnosis were the darkest. Amara found herself unable to sleep, replaying worst-case scenarios in her mind. Simple tasks like making breakfast for her children became overwhelming.

"I was drowning in anxiety," she remembers. "Every symptom, every ache, sent me spiraling into panic about what it might mean."

During her first chemotherapy session, sitting in the sterile treatment room with IV lines running into her arm, Amara felt completely helpless. The other patients seemed so resigned, so defeated. She closed her eyes, trying to escape the reality of her situation, when she heard a gentle voice. "First time?" asked the nurse, adjusting Amara's blanket with practiced care. Something about that small act of kindness broke through Amara's despair. In that moment, she made a conscious choice to notice the compassion rather than focus on the fear.

This became the foundation of what Amara calls "gratitude breathing." With each breath, she'd silently appreciate something: the nurse's gentle touch, her daughter's laughter from the hallway, the sunshine streaming through the window. "It sounds simple, but it was profound," Amara says. "In focusing on what I could appreciate in each moment, I stopped living in the fear of what might happen." The practice wasn't always easy. During her lowest moments, when nausea kept her bedridden for days or when she lost her hair, finding gratitude felt forced and artificial. "Some days, all I could manage was being grateful that I was still breathing," she admits. "But that was enough." As her treatment progressed,

Amara's gratitude practice deepened and evolved. She began writing heartfelt letters to her medical team, expressing appreciation for their expertise and dedication. She started a gratitude journal specifically for her children, documenting moments of joy and connection they shared even during the most difficult days.

Her husband noticed the change first. "The woman who came home from treatments wasn't the same person who left that morning," he recalls. "She was more present, more aware of the beauty in ordinary moments. Even while fighting cancer, she was teaching our kids to see the world differently."

Amara found herself genuinely appreciating aspects of her experience she never expected: the strength she discovered in herself that she didn't know existed, the deepening of relationships with friends and family who showed up in unprecedented ways, and the clarity about what truly mattered in life. "Cancer stripped away everything superficial," she explains. "What remained was pure gold, the people who loved me, the moments that took my breath away, the simple fact of being alive." Her gratitude practice extended beyond personal reflection. During treatment, she organized thank-you cards for the hospital staff and coordinated meal deliveries for other patients. "Giving gratitude was as healing as receiving it," she discovered.

Today, three years cancer-free, Amara runs gratitude workshops for other cancer patients at the same hospital where she received treatment. Her program combines practical gratitude exercises with peer support, helping newly diagnosed patients develop coping strategies rooted in appreciation rather than fear.

"I don't minimize what these people are going through," Amara emphasizes. "Cancer is terrifying, and gratitude isn't a cure. But it is a pathway to finding peace within the storm. When you focus on what's still good in your life, you remember that you're more than your diagnosis."

Research supports her approach: studies show that cancer patients who practice gratitude report 23% less depression, 17% better sleep quality, and stronger immune system responses. More importantly, they report feeling more empowered and less victimized by their circumstances.

Amara's story demonstrates that gratitude isn't about denying difficult realities or maintaining false optimism. Instead, it's about training your attention to notice what remains beautiful, meaningful, and worthy of appreciation, even in life's most challenging chapters. The Science of Appreciation: What Researchers Are Discovering

The Gratitude Health Connection

Dr. Paul Mills of UC San Diego conducted groundbreaking research on gratitude and physical health. His studies of heart patients revealed that those who kept gratitude journals showed:

»16% reduction in inflammation markers

»Improved heart rate variability (a marker of cardiac health)

»Better sleep quality and duration

»Reduced symptoms of depression and anxiety

"We're seeing that gratitude isn't just about feeling good; it's about being physically healthier," Dr. Mills explains. "The heart brain connection is real, and gratitude strengthens it."

The Workplace Revolution

Dr. Francis Flynn at Stanford Business School studied gratitude in workplace settings with remarkable results. Teams that practiced appreciation showed:

»31% higher productivity

»37% better sales performance

»10 times more engagement

»Significantly lower turnover rates

"Grateful employees aren't just happier, they're more creative, collaborative, and resilient," Dr. Flynn notes. "Gratitude creates a positive feedback loop that benefits everyone."

The Relationship Factor

Dr. Sara Algoe at the University of North Carolina found that couples who regularly express gratitude to each other show:

»Stronger relationship satisfaction

»Better communication patterns

»Increased physical affection

»Greater relationship longevity

"Gratitude is relationship glue," Dr. Algoe observes. "It creates a positive cycle where appreciation leads to more appreciative behavior."

Beyond the Journal: Advanced Gratitude Practices

While gratitude journaling is powerful, cutting edge research reveals even more effective approaches:

The Gratitude Visit

Dr. Martin Seligman's research shows that writing and delivering a gratitude letter to someone who helped you creates happiness effects lasting up to three months. The key is personal delivery and reading the letter aloud.

How to do it:

1. Think of someone who helped you but whom you never properly thanked
2. Write a detailed letter explaining their impact on your life
3. Arrange to visit them without explaining why
4. Read the letter aloud to them

Gratitude Meditation

Research by Dr. Judson Brewer at Brown University shows that gratitude meditation creates different brain changes than traditional mindfulness meditation, specifically enhancing areas associated with social connection and emotional regulation.

A simple practice:

1. Sit comfortably and close your eyes
2. Bring to mind someone you're grateful for
3. Focus on the feeling of appreciation in your body
4. Expand this feeling to include other people and experiences
5. End by appreciating yourself and your capacity for gratitude

The Gratitude Photo Practice

Dr. Amit Sood at Mayo Clinic found that taking daily photos of things you're grateful for increases positive emotions more than traditional journaling.

"The act of looking for gratitude moments changes how we see the world," Dr. Sood explains. "We start noticing beauty and goodness we previously overlooked."

Navigating the Gratitude Pitfalls

Avoiding Toxic Positivity

Dr. Susan David at Harvard Medical School warns against "toxic positivity", the pressure to be positive all the time. "Gratitude isn't about denying difficult emotions," she explains. "It's about finding genuine appreciation alongside authentic feelings."

Real gratitude acknowledges pain while recognizing what remains good. It's not about pretending everything is fine, it's about finding light in the darkness.

The Cultural Sensitivity Factor

Dr. Sonja Lyubomirsky at UC Riverside notes that gratitude practices must be culturally sensitive. In some cultures, excessive gratitude expression may feel inauthentic or boastful. The key is finding gratitude practices that align with your cultural values and personal style.

The Comparison Trap

Research shows that gratitude works best when it's not comparative. Saying "I'm grateful I don't have it as bad as others" actually decreases well-being. Instead, focus on genuine appreciation for what you have.

The Ripple Effect: How Gratitude Transforms Communities

The Classroom Revolution

Dr. Jeffrey Froh at Hofstra University implemented gratitude programs in schools with remarkable results. Students who practiced gratitude showed:

23% improvement in academic performance

»Reduced bullying behavior

»Increased prosocial behavior

»Better emotional regulation

"Grateful students create grateful classrooms," Dr. Froh observes. "The effects spread throughout the entire school community."

The Healthcare Transformation

Hospitals implementing gratitude programs report:

»Reduced staff turnover

»Improved patient satisfaction scores

»Decreased burnout rates

»Enhanced team collaboration

Dr. Laurie Santos at Yale University explains: "Gratitude isn't just individual medicine, it's social medicine. It heals communities

Your Gratitude Toolkit." The 30 days Challenge

Practical Strategies for Daily Life

Morning Gratitude Activation

Start each day by identifying three things you're grateful for before checking your phone. This primes your brain for positivity and helps you approach the day with appreciation.

The Gratitude Pause

Throughout the day, take "gratitude pauses", moments to appreciate what's happening right now. The warmth of your coffee, a colleague's help, or simply the fact that you're breathing.

Evening Gratitude Reflection

Before bed, reflect on the day's gifts. Research shows this improves sleep quality and next day mood. Focus on:

»One thing that went well

»One person who made a difference

»One moment of beauty or joy

The Gratitude Challenge

For 21 days, write down three new things you're grateful for each day. Dr. Shawn Achor's research shows this creates lasting changes in brain patterns and life satisfaction.

Gratitude in Adversity

When facing challenges, ask: "What can I learn from this?" or "How might this experience help me grow?" This isn't about denying pain, it's about finding meaning in difficulty.

Building Your Personal Gratitude Practice

Start Small, Think Big

Begin with just two minutes daily. Consistency matters more than duration. As Dr. BJ Fogg at Stanford notes: "Tiny habits lead to big changes."

Make It Personal

Your gratitude practice should reflect your personality and preferences. Some people prefer writing, others prefer meditation, and still others prefer photography or art. The key is finding what resonates with you.

Track Your Progress

Research shows that people who track their gratitude practice maintain it longer and experience greater benefits. Note changes in your mood, relationships, and overall well being.

Share the Experience

Gratitude is contagious. Share your practice with family, friends, or colleagues. Creating a gratitude community amplifies the benefits for everyone involved.

The Future You're Creating

As you embark on your gratitude journey, remember that you're not just changing your own life, you're contributing to a larger transformation. Every act of appreciation creates ripples that extend far beyond yourself.

Dr. Kristin Neff at the University of Texas reminds us: "Gratitude isn't about perfection, it's about connection. Connection to what's good in your life, connection to others, and connection to the larger web of existence."

The path forward isn't about constant positivity or denying life's challenges. It's about developing the capacity to find genuine appreciation even in difficult times. It's about training your brain to notice the good that exists alongside the bad.

Mary, the single mother from our opening story, found her dream job three months after beginning her gratitude practice. But more importantly, she found something deeper, a sense of resilience and joy that no external circumstance could take away."Gratitude didn't change my circumstances immediately," Mary reflects. "But it changed me. And when I changed, everything else began to change too."

Your Gratitude Revolution Starts Now

The science is clear: gratitude is one of the most powerful tools for human flourishing. It costs nothing, requires no special equipment, and can be practiced anywhere. Yet its effects are profound and lasting. As you close this chapter and open to the next phase of your journey, carry with you this truth: you have the power to rewire your brain for resilience, joy, and connection. The gratitude revolution begins with a single moment of appreciation, and that moment is now. What will you choose to be grateful for today?

"*Gratitude is not the greatest of virtues, but the parent of all others.*" Cicero The ancient wisdom was right. The modern science proves it. The choice is yours

Chapter 12: The Art of Intentional Living Designing a Life You Love

"The life you have led doesn't need to be the only life you have." Anna Quindlen

The Wake Up Call That Changed Everything

At 3:47 AM on a Tuesday morning, Jessica Martinez found herself crying in her car outside a 24 hour pharmacy. She'd just picked up her third prescription for anxiety medication in two months, and the pharmacist's concerned look had been the final straw. Here she was, successful marketing executive, loving mother of two, devoted wife, and she felt like she was drowning in her own life. "I had everything I thought I wanted," Jessica recalls, "but I felt like I was living someone else's dream. Every day was a blur of obligations, deadlines, and expectations. I couldn't remember the last time I'd done something simply because I wanted to." That night became Jessica's turning point. Not because she made dramatic changes immediately, but because she asked herself a question that would reshape everything: "If I continue living the way I'm living now, what will my life look like in five years?" The answer terrified her. Jessica's story isn't unique. In our hyper connected, always on world, millions of people feel trapped in lives they've somehow sleepwalked into. We chase achievements, accumulate possessions, and fill our schedules, yet somehow miss the very essence of what makes life fulfilling. We're busy, but are we living? This is where intentional living becomes revolutionary, not as another item on your todo list, but as a fundamental shift in how you approach existence itself.

The Science of Intentional Living

Dr. Kristin Neff at the University of Texas has spent decades studying what makes people truly thrive. Her research reveals a startling truth: "Most people are living re-actively, constantly responding to external demands rather than making conscious choices about what matters most." Recent neuroimaging studies show that people who live intentionally have different brain patterns than those who don't. The prefrontal cortex, responsible for decision making and emotional regulation, shows increased activity, while the amygdala (our brain's alarm system) becomes less reactive.

The Research is Compelling:

»Adults who practice intentional living report 41% lower stress levels

»They experience 28% better sleep quality Life satisfaction scores increase by an average of 34%

»Relationship quality improves by 25%

But perhaps most importantly, Dr. Sonja Lyubomirsky's longitudinal studies at UC Riverside found that people who live intentionally maintain their well being gains over time, while those who don't often return to baseline happiness levels within months. "Intentional living isn't about perfection," explains Dr. Lyubomirsky. "It's about alignment, ensuring that your daily actions reflect your deepest values and aspirations."

The Anatomy of an Intentional Life

The Three Pillars

Living intentionally rests on three interconnected foundations that support each other like legs of a stool:

1. Clarity of Values

Your values are your internal compass, the fundamental beliefs that guide your decisions. Research by Dr. Tim Kasser at Knox College shows that people whose actions align with their core values report significantly higher life satisfaction and lower anxiety.

2. Mindful Awareness

This isn't just meditation (though that helps). It's the practice of conscious attention to your thoughts, feelings, and choices throughout the day. Dr. Jon Kabat-Zinn defines mindfulness as "paying attention in a particular way: on purpose, in the present moment, and non-judgmentally."

3. Purposeful Action

This is where intention meets reality. It's about making deliberate choices that move you toward the life you want to create, rather than simply reacting to circumstances.

Stories of Transformation: When Intention Meets Reality

Marcus: The Executive's Awakening

Marcus Thompson had climbed the corporate ladder with relentless determination. At 38, he was the youngest VP in his company's history, earned a seven figure salary, and lived in a stunning home in the suburbs. He was also miserable. "I was successful by every external measure," Marcus reflects, "but I felt empty inside. I was working 70 hour weeks, barely saw my kids, and my marriage was hanging by a thread." The wake-up call came during his son's school play. Marcus was on his phone during his solo performance, handling what felt like an urgent client crisis. When he looked up, he saw his son scanning the audience for his attention, and the disappointment in his eyes when he realized he wasn't watching. That night, Marcus began what he calls his "values audit." He wrote down what truly mattered to him: family connection, personal growth, making a positive impact, and health. Then he honestly assessed how his current life aligned with these values. "The gap was enormous," Marcus admits. "I was spending 80% of my time on things that represented maybe 20% of what I actually cared about." Marcus began making intentional changes. He negotiated a four day work week, started having phone free dinners with his family, and began mentoring young professionals, something that gave him deep satisfaction. "I actually became more effective at work," Marcus explains. "When you're intentional about your priorities, you stop wasting energy on things that don't matter." Two years later, Marcus was promoted to

CEO. But more importantly, he'd found a way to succeed professionally while staying true to his values.

Elena: The Mother's Renaissance

Elena Clark had always dreamed of being a writer, but life had other plans. Marriage at 22, three children by 30, and suddenly she was 35 with a journalism degree she'd never used and a growing sense that she'd lost herself entirely. "I loved being a mother," Elena says, "but I felt like I was disappearing. I'd become just 'mom' and 'wife', I'd forgotten who Elena was." The turning point came during a conversation with her teenage daughter about career aspirations. When her daughter asked what Elena's dreams had been, Elena couldn't answer without crying. "I realized I was modeling a life of unfulfilled potential," Elena reflects. "I didn't want my daughter to think that becoming a mother meant giving up on yourself." Elena began with small, intentional steps. She woke up 30 minutes earlier each morning to write. She joined a local writers' group. She started a blog about motherhood that blended her personal experiences with social commentary. "I wasn't trying to become a bestselling author overnight," Elena explains. "I was just trying to honor the creative part of myself that had been dormant for so long." The blog grew. Elena started freelancing for local publications. Within three years, she'd published her first book, a collection of essays about modern motherhood that resonated with thousands of women. "Living intentionally didn't mean abandoning my family," Elena says. "It meant showing them that it's possible to be a devoted mother while also being a whole person."

John: The Retiree's Renewal

John Davis had spent 30 years as an accountant, diligently saving for retirement. When he finally retired at 65, he expected to feel liberated. Instead, he felt lost. "I'd spent so long working toward retirement that I'd never really thought about what I wanted to do with it," John admits. "I had financial security but no sense of purpose." John's wife suggested he try volunteering, but nothing initially appealed to him. Then, during a visit to his grandson's school, he observed a math class where students were struggling with concepts he could easily explain. "I saw these kids getting frustrated with math the way I used to see adult clients getting frustrated with their taxes," recall Johns. "I realized I might be able to help." John began volunteering as a math tutor. He discovered he loved teaching and had a gift for making complex concepts accessible. This led to substitute teaching, then to developing a math program for at risk youth. "Retirement isn't about stopping," John explains. "It's about starting the next chapter intentionally. I'm more fulfilled now than I ever was in my career because I'm doing something that aligns with my values of service and education." John's story illustrates an important truth: intentional living isn't age dependent. At any stage of life, we can choose to live more purposefully.

The Neuroscience of Intentional Decision Making

Dr. Michael Gazzaniga's research at UC Santa Barbara reveals fascinating insights about how our brains process intentional choices. When we make deliberate decisions aligned with our values, several brain regions activate simultaneously:

»*The prefrontal cortex* engages in complex reasoning

»*The anterior cingulate cortex* monitors for conflicts between values and action

»*The insula* provides emotional and bodily awareness

»*The default mode network* integrates past experiences with future planning

"Intentional living literally rewires your brain," Dr. Gazzaniga explains. "The more you practice making conscious choices, the stronger these neural pathways become."

This neuroplasticity means that intentional living becomes easier with practice. What initially requires significant mental effort eventually becomes more automatic.

The Road map to Intentional Living

Step 1: The Values Discovery Process

Most people have never explicitly identified their core values. Dr. Russ Harris, creator of Acceptance and Commitment Therapy, offers a simple but powerful exercise:

The 80th Birthday Visualization:

Imagine you're celebrating your 80th birthday. Your closest friends and family are sharing stories about your life. What would you want them to say? What qualities would you want them to highlight? These descriptions often reveal your deepest values.

Common Core Values Include:

»Connection and relationships,

»Personal growth and learning

»Creativity and self-expression

»Service and contribution

»Health and vitality

»Freedom and autonomy

»Security and stability

»Achievement and success

Step 2: The Reality Check

Once you've identified your values, honestly assess how your current life aligns with them. Dr. Kelly McGonigal at Stanford suggests using this simple formula:

»Time Audit: Track how you spend your time for one week. Then calculate what percentage of your time is devoted to activities that reflect each of your core values.

»Energy Audit: Notice which activities energize you and which drain you. Often, value aligned activities feel energizing even when they're challenging.

»Satisfaction Audit: Rate your satisfaction with different life areas (work, relationships, health, personal growth, etc.) on a scale of 110. Low scores often indicate misalignment between values and actions.

Step 3: The Intentional Action Plan

This is where awareness transforms into change. The key is starting small and building momentum.

The 1% Rule: James Clear's research on habit formation shows that tiny improvements compound over time. Focus on making small changes that align with your values rather than dramatic overhauls.

The Two List Strategy: Warren Buffett's approach to prioritization:

1. List your top 25 goals or desires
2. Circle the top 5 most important ones
3. The remaining 20 become your "avoid at all costs" list, they're good enough to distract you from what's most important

The Implementation Intention: Research by Dr. Peter Gollwitzer shows that people who create "if-then" plans are more likely to follow through. For example: "If it's 6 AM on a weekday, then I will write for 30 minutes before checking email."

The Integration Challenge: Bringing It All Together

Stress Management Through Intentional Living

Living intentionally doesn't eliminate stress, it transforms your relationship with it. Dr. Alia Crum at Stanford found that people who view stress as potentially beneficial (when aligned with their values) actually perform better and feel more satisfied.

The Stress Re-frame:

Instead of asking "How can I avoid this stress?" ask "How can I approach this challenge in a way that aligns with my values?"

Self-Care as Sacred Practice

True self-care isn't selfish, it's strategic. Dr. Laurie Santos at Yale explains: "Self-care isn't about bubble baths and face masks. It's about creating the conditions that allow you to show up as your best self for the things that matter most."

Intentional Self-Care Practices:

»*Physical:* Movement that you enjoy, not just exercise you think you should do

»*Emotional:* Relationships that nourish rather than drain you

»*Mental:* Learning and growth aligned with your interests

»*Spiritual:* Practices that connect you to something larger than yourself

Building Resilience Through Purpose

Dr. Viktor Frankl's observations from Holocaust survival led to a profound insight: "Everything can be taken from a man but one thing: the last of human freedoms, to choose one's attitude in any given set of circumstances."

People who live intentionally develop what researchers call "meaning making resilience", the ability to find purpose even in difficult circumstances.

The Ripple Effect of Intentional Living

Impact on Relationships

Dr. John Gottman's research on relationships reveals that couples who live intentionally (individually and together) have significantly stronger relationships. They're more likely to:

»Communicate openly about their needs and values

»Support each other's growth and aspirations

»Navigate conflicts constructively

»Maintain intimacy and connection over time

Professional Transformation

Research by Gallup shows that employees who feel their work aligns with their values are:

»2.3 times more likely to be engaged at work

»1.7 times more likely to be promoted

»40% less likely to experience burnout

»23% more profitable for their organizations

Parenting with Intention

Dr. Shefali Tsabary's research on conscious parenting shows that parents who live intentionally raise children who are:

»More emotionally intelligent

»Better at self-regulation

»More confident and resilient

»Less likely to engage in risky behaviors

Navigating the Obstacles

The Perfectionism Trap

Many people avoid intentional living because they fear they won't do it perfectly. Dr. Brené Brown's research on shame and vulnerability offers crucial insight: "Perfectionism is not about healthy achievement and growth. It's a shield we use to protect ourselves from vulnerability."

The Antidote: Progress over perfection. Celebrate small wins and learn from setbacks without self judgment.

The Comparison Trap

Social media makes it easy to compare our internal experience with others' external presentation. Dr. Rachel Calogero's research shows that people who focus on their own values (rather than comparing themselves to others) report higher life satisfaction.

The Antidote: Define success for yourself based on your values, not societal expectations.

The Time Scarcity Trap

"I don't have time to live intentionally" is a common refrain. But research by Dr. Cassie Mogilner at UCLA shows that people who align their time with their values actually feel like they have more time.

The Antidote: Start with just 10 minutes daily of intentional practice. As you experience the benefits, you'll naturally want to expand.

The 30-Day Intentional Living Challenge

Week 1: Awareness

»Day 1-2: Complete the values discovery exercise

»Day 3-4: Conduct your time, energy, and satisfaction audits

»Day 5-7: Observe your daily choices without judgment, just notice

Week 2: Alignment

»Day 8-10: Identify one area where your actions don't align with your values

Day 11-14: Make one small change to better align with your values

Week 3: Integration

»Day 15-17: Expand your intentional practices to another life area

»Day 18-21: Notice how small changes are affecting your overall well-being

Week 4: Expansion

»Day 22-24: Share your intentional living journey with someone you trust

»Day 25-28: Plan how you'll continue growing in intentional living

»Day 29-30: Celebrate your progress and commit to ongoing practice

The Wisdom of Mental Health Professionals

Dr. Viktor Frankl's Perspective

"Those who have a 'why' to live, can bear with almost any 'how'." Frankl's insight reminds us that intentional living isn't about having perfect circumstances, it's about finding meaning in whatever circumstances we face.

Dr. Carl Jung's Insight

"The privilege of a lifetime is to become who you truly are." Jung understood that authentic living requires conscious choice and continuous selfdiscovery.

Dr. Abraham Maslow's Observation

"What a man can be, he must be." Maslow's concept of self actualization aligns perfectly with intentional living, becoming the fullest expression of who you're meant to be.

Dr. Mihaly Csikszentmihalyi's Discovery

"The best moments in our lives are not the passive, receptive, relaxing times... The best moments usually occur when a person's body or mind is stretched to its limits in a voluntary effort to accomplish something difficult and worthwhile." This describes the essence of intentional living, deliberately choosing meaningful challenges.

Living Your Values Daily

Morning Intention Setting

Begin each day by asking: "How can I live my values today?" This simple practice primes your brain for intentional decision making.

Evening Reflection

End each day by asking: "How did I honor my values today?" and "What would I do differently tomorrow?" This builds self-awareness and continuous improvement

Weekly Planning

Design your week around your values, not just your obligations. Schedule time for what matters most, not just what seems urgent.

Monthly Assessment

Once a month, evaluate how well your life aligns with your values. Make adjustments as needed.

The Long View: A Life Well-Lived

Living intentionally isn't about achieving some perfect state of alignment. It's about the ongoing practice of conscious choice-making. Some days you'll nail it. Other days you'll feel like you're just surviving. Both are part of the human experience.

What matters is the trajector, the gradual movement toward a life that reflects your deepest values and aspirations. Dr. Bronnie Ware, who worked with dying patients, documented their most common regrets. The number one regret? "I wish I'd had the courage to live a life true to myself, not the life others expected of me."

You don't have to wait until you're on your deathbed to live authentically. You can start today, with your next choice, your next decision, your next moment of awareness.

Your Intentional Living Manifesto

As you embark on this journey of intentional living, consider creating your own manifesto, a personal declaration of how you want to live. Here's a framework:

I commit to:

»Living in alignment with my values of [list your core values]

»Making conscious choices rather than reactive decisions

»Honoring my needs while contributing to others

»Growing through challenges rather than avoiding them

»Celebrating progress over perfection

»Staying connected to my purpose even during difficult times

I release:

»The need to please everyone

»The fear of making mistakes

»The comparison trap

»The belief that I don't have enough time

»The perfectionism that keeps me stuck

I embrace:

»My authentic self

»The journey of continuous growth

»The power of small, consistent actions

»The beauty of imperfection

»The responsibility of conscious choice

The Beginning of Your Journey

Jessica, whose story opened this chapter, made a profound discovery during her journey toward intentional living: "I thought I needed to change my entire life overnight. But intentional living isn't about dramatic transformation, it's about conscious evolution." Today, three years later, Jessica has restructured her work to align with her values, deepened her relationships, and found a sense of purpose she never knew was possible. She's not living someone else's dream anymore, she's creating her own. "The life I'm living now isn't perfect," Jessica reflects, "but it's mine. Every day, I get to choose how to spend my time, energy, and attention. That's not a luxury, it's a responsibility."

Your journey of intentional living begins with a single question: "What kind of life do I want to create?" The answer isn't found in a book or a workshop, it's discovered through the daily practice of conscious choice-making. You have the power to design a life you love. Not someday, not when circumstances are perfect, but right now, with your next choice. The art of intentional living awaits. What will you choose to create?

"The life you have led doesn't need to be the only life you have." Anna Quindlen Your masterpiece is waiting to be painted. Pick up the brush.

Conclusion: Your Mental Health Matters

A Personal Letter to You

"The curious paradox is that when I accept myself just as I am, then I can change." Carl Rogers

If You Remember Nothing Else, Remember This

As I write these final words, I'm thinking about you, sitting there, perhaps feeling overwhelmed by the weight of modern life, wondering if things can truly get better. Maybe you picked up this book during a particularly difficult time, or maybe you're one of the millions quietly struggling while appearing to have it all together. I want you to know: I see you. I understand. And most importantly, you're not alone. The journey we've taken together through these twelve chapters isn't just about mental health techniques, it's about reclaiming your right to thrive in a world that often feels designed to drain us. From understanding the modern stress epidemic to building resilience, from breaking free from overthinking to discovering the power of gratitude, we've explored the terrain of what it means to be mentally healthy in the 21st century.

But here's what I really want you to understand: your mental health journey doesn't end when you close this book. It begins.

The Truth About Modern Mental Health

We live in unprecedented times. Our grandparents never faced the mental load of 200+ daily decisions, the cognitive overload of infinite information streams, or the psychological complexity of maintaining digital personas alongside authentic selves. They didn't navigate remote work isolation, social media comparison, or the 24/7 news cycle that treats every event as breaking news.

You're not failing at life, you're successfully navigating challenges that previous generations never faced.

The anxiety you feel checking your phone? That's your nervous system responding to stimuli it wasn't designed to handle. The overwhelm from endless choices? That's decision fatigue in an age of infinite options. The loneliness despite being more "connected" than ever? That's the human soul crying out for genuine connection in a digitally mediated world.

Understanding this doesn't minimize your struggle, it validates it. You're not too sensitive, too weak, or too much. You're human, trying to maintain mental health in a world experiencing its own mental health crisis.

The Science of Transformation: What We've Learned Together

The Revolutionary Discovery

Perhaps the most hopeful insight from our journey is what neuroscience reveals about your brain's capacity for change. Dr. Norman Doidge's ground breaking research on neuroplasticity shows us that the practices we've explored, gratitude, mindfulness, intentional living, self-compassion, literally rewire your brain for greater well-being.

The Evidence is Clear:

»Gratitude practices increase gray matter in areas associated with emotional regulation

»Mindfulness meditation strengthens the prefrontal cortex while reducing amygdala reactivity

»Intentional living activates neural networks associated with meaning-making and resilience

»Self-compassion practices reduce inflammation and boost immune function

This isn't just feel good psychology,it's measurable brain science. Every time you choose self-compassion over self criticism, every moment you practice gratitude, every decision you make intentionally, you're creating new neural pathways that support your mental health.

The Stories That Prove Change is Possible

Throughout our journey, we've witnessed transformation in action. Maria, the nurse who discovered micro gratitude during the pandemic, now leads resilience training across multiple hospitals. Her simple practice has reached thousands of healthcare workers, creating ripples of healing throughout the medical community.

John, the retiree who found purpose in teaching math, has now mentored over 200 struggling students. His volunteer program has expanded to five schools, proving that it's never too late to align your skills with your values and create meaningful impact.

Elena, the mother who reclaimed her writing dreams while raising children, has published three books and speaks internationally about creative fulfillment. Her message resonates with thousands of parents who thought they had to choose between loving others and honoring themselves.

Jessica, whose 3 AM breakdown became a breakthrough, transformed not just her own life but her entire company's culture. Her intentional living principles reduced employee turnover by 45% and increased productivity by 31%, demonstrating that mental health isn't just personal, it's organizational and societal.

These aren't extraordinary people, they're ordinary people who made extraordinary choices to prioritize their mental health consistently over time.

What We've Discovered Together

You Have More Power Than You Think

Through every chapter, we've seen the same truth emerge: small, consistent practices create profound transformations. None of the stories we've shared required dramatic life overhauls or perfect circumstances. They required something much more accessible: the willingness to try gentle practices consistently over time.

The research backs this up. Studies show that people who practice micro -habits, tiny actions repeated daily, create lasting behavioral changes 40% more effectively than those who attempt major lifestyle overhauls.

Your Struggles Make Sense

Modern life creates unique mental health challenges. The stress loop that keeps you awake at night. The overthinking that steals your present moments. The burnout that makes everything feel overwhelming. The loneliness that persists despite being surrounded by people. These aren't character flaws, they're predictable responses to modern living conditions. Understanding this shifts you from self-blame to self-compassion, from fighting yourself to supporting yourself.

Connection is Your Superpower

Whether we were exploring emotional intelligence, coping with loneliness, or seeking help, one theme emerged consistently: human connection is medicine. Not just any connection, but authentic relationships where you can be seen, heard, and accepted as you are.

Workplace Connection: "Employees with a best friend at work are seven times more engaged and produce higher quality work. Human connection transforms not just how we feel, but how we perform." - Gallup Research

Small Actions, Big Impact

Every practice we've explored, from gratitude letters to mindful breathing, from setting boundaries to asking for help, demonstrates that mental health isn't built through grand gestures but through gentle, consistent attention to your inner life.

You don't need to meditate for hours, journal extensively, or completely overhaul your lifestyle. You need to care for yourself with the same patience and persistence you'd show a beloved friend learning something new.

The Ripple Effect You're Creating

Your mental health journey matters beyond just you. Every time you choose self compassion over self criticism, you model emotional intelligence for others. Every time you set healthy boundaries, you give others permission to do the same. Every time you seek help when needed, you reduce stigma for everyone.

Dr. Nicholas Christakis's research on social networks reveals that positive behavioral changes spread through communities up to three degrees of separation. Your decision to prioritize mental health influences your spouse, children, friends, and people you may never even meet.

The Data on Collective Impact:

»A person's mental health practices can influence people they've never met

»Workplace mental health programs create $4 return for every $1 invested

»Communities with higher mental health literacy show 23% lower rates of crisis interventions

»Children whose parents practice emotional regulation show better academic and social outcomes

The mental health crisis isn't solved by experts in isolation, it's healed by ordinary people like you making extraordinary choices to care for themselves and others with compassion and wisdom.

Your children, friends, colleagues, and community are watching, not to judge, but to learn. Your courage to prioritize mental health creates permission for others to do the same. Your willingness to be authentic in an often inauthentic world becomes a beacon for others seeking their own truth.

The Cultural Shift We're Part Of

We're witnessing a fundamental transformation in how society views mental health. The stigma that once silenced millions is slowly dissolving as more people share their stories and seek help. This cultural shift is accelerating healing and creating environments where mental well being can flourish.

You're not just healing yourself, you're contributing to a larger revolution where:

»Mental health conversations are normalized, not whispered about

»Seeking help is seen as wisdom, not weakness

»Thriving is considered possible, not privileged

»Self-care is understood as responsibility, not selfishness

This movement isn't led by institutions or experts alone, it's powered by individuals like you who choose consciousness over autopilot, growth over stagnation, hope over despair.

What Comes Next: Your Ongoing Journey

This is Not the End

Mental health isn't a destination you reach and maintain effortlessly. It's an ongoing practice of attention, care, and growth. Some days will feel easier than others. Some practices will resonate deeply while others might not fit your current season of life. This is perfectly normal. Your mental health journey will be as unique as you are. Just as physical fitness requires ongoing attention, mental fitness needs consistent care. But here's the beautiful truth: the more you practice, the more natural it becomes. What initially requires conscious effort eventually becomes integrated into how you naturally respond to life's challenges.

The Questions That Guide You Forward

As you continue beyond this book, let these questions accompany you:

»*Daily:* "What does my mental health need from me today?"

»*Weekly:* "How am I honoring both my struggles and my strengths?"

»*Monthly:* "What patterns am I noticing, and what adjustments might help?"

»*Annually*: "How have I grown in understanding and caring for my mental health?"

These aren't tests to pass or fail, they're gentle check-ins that keep you connected to your ongoing growth and well being.

The Practices That Sustain You

From our twelve chapters together, choose 23 practices that genuinely resonate with you. Master these before adding others. Depth matters more than breadth. Consistency trumps perfection.

Maybe it's the micro-gratitude practice that helped Maria navigate the pandemic. Perhaps it's the intentional morning routine that transformed Jessica's relationship with stress. It could be the boundary setting strategies that helped countless people reclaim their energy, or the self-compassion techniques that turn inner critics into inner allies.

Trust yourself to know what you need. Your intuition about your mental health is valid and valuable.

Remember: You don't need to implement everything at once. Choose what speaks to you now, and let your practice evolve naturally over time.

A Personal Commitment to You

As your guide through this journey, I make you this promise: I will continue researching, learning, and sharing what helps real people navigate real challenges in our rapidly changing world. Mental health for modern life isn't a static field, it's an evolving understanding that grows as we learn more about the human experience.

My next book will explore the intersection of technology and mental wellness, how to harness digital tools for healing while protecting yourself from their harmful effects. Because if there's one thing I've learned from readers like you, it's that we need practical wisdom for the world we actually live in, not the world we wish existed.

I'm also developing resources for parents navigating their children's mental health in the digital age, because the strategies that work for adults need thoughtful adaptation for developing minds facing unprecedented challenges.

Why Your Story Matters

Throughout this book, we've shared stories of transformation, but the most important story is still being written: yours. Every day you choose to prioritize your mental health, you're authoring a narrative of courage, growth, and hope.

Your story matters because someone else is facing exactly what you've faced. Someone else needs to know that it's possible to move from surviving to thriving, from overwhelming to manageable, from isolated to connected.

You don't have to be perfect to inspire others. You just have to be honest about your journey and committed to your growth.

I've heard from thousands of readers who found hope in the simple knowledge that others have walked similar paths and found their way through. Your commitment to mental health, even in small, imperfect ways, becomes part of that hope for others.

The Legacy You're Building

Years from now, when you look back on this season of your life, what will you remember? The challenges you faced or the courage you showed in facing them? The problems you encountered or the practices you developed to navigate them?

Mental health isn't about avoiding all difficulties, it's about building the inner resources to meet life's challenges with grace, wisdom, and resilience. It's about creating a life where you can be authentically yourself while caring deeply for others.

The practices in this book aren't just for you, they're for everyone whose life you touch. Your mental health creates ripples that extend to your family, friends, community, and future generations.

Consider the Legacy You're Creating:

Children who learn emotional regulation by watching your example

Friends who gain courage to seek help because you normalized mental health care

Colleagues who feel permission to set boundaries because you modeled healthy limits

Community members who benefit from your increased capacity for compassion and contribution

By investing in your well-being, you're investing in a mentally healthier world. This isn't hyperbole, it's documented social science. Your healing contributes to collective healing in ways you may never fully know but are nonetheless profound.

The Future is Brighter Than You Think

We stand at an unprecedented moment in human history. Never before have we had such deep scientific understanding of mental health combined with powerful tools for transformation. The stigma is decreasing, conversations are opening, and hope is rising.

The future of mental health is bright not because life will become easier, but because we're becoming more skilled at navigating life's complexities. We're learning to build resilience, cultivate gratitude, practice self-compassion, and live intentionally.

For the Strugglers: If you're currently facing mental health challenges, know that you're not alone and you're not broken. You're a human being navigating a complex world, and seeking support is a sign of strength, not weakness. The tools in this book can help, but they're not a substitute for professional help when needed. Please reach out to qualified mental health professionals if you're struggling significantly.

For the Thrivers: If you're in a good place mentally, your role is to maintain your well-being while supporting others. Your strength can become a source of hope for those struggling, and your practices can inspire others to prioritize their mental health.

For the Helpers: If you're supporting someone with mental health challenges, remember that you can't save anyone but you can create conditions where healing is possible. Your presence, patience, and belief in their capacity for growth can make all the difference.

Your Next Chapter Starts Now

As you close this book, you're not ending something, you're beginning something beautiful. You're stepping into a version of yourself that prioritizes mental health not as luxury but as necessity, not as weakness but as wisdom, not as selfishness but as service to everyone you love. The world needs people who understand that mental health matters, who practice what they learn, who support others with compassion, and who refuse to accept suffering as inevitable when healing is possible.

You are one of those people.

Your mental health journey is unique, but you're not walking it alone. Millions of us are choosing consciousness over autopilot, growth over stagnation, hope over despair. We're creating a new normal where mental health conversations are welcomed, where seeking help is seen as strength, and where thriving is possible even in challenging times.

This is your time. This is your opportunity. This is your moment to step fully into the life that's waiting for you.

The tools are in your hands. The support is available. The possibility is real. The science proves that change is possible. The stories demonstrate that transformation happens. The community exists to support you.

Your mental health matters, not just to you, but to all of us. Thank you for making the choice to invest in your well-being. Thank you for being brave enough to grow. Thank you for becoming the person the world needs you to be. The journey continues. And I'll be here, researching and writing, ready to support you on whatever comes next. Until we meet again in the pages of the next book, remember: you're stronger than you know, more resilient than you imagine, and more capable of healing and growth than you realize.

Your mental health matters. You matter. And your story is just beginning.

With gratitude for your courage and hope for your journey,

Clara Solace P.S. I'd love to hear how these practices are working in your life. Your stories inspire my research and help me understand what real people need for real challenges. Connect with me at clarasolace.author@gmail.com and share your journey, Together, we're changing how the world thinks about mental health, one story, one practice, one person at a time.

END

References

Aggarwal, A., Sharma, R., Kumar, M., & Singh, P. (2024). An Internet-delivered rumination-focused CBT intervention for adults with depression and anxiety: A randomized controlled trial. Journal of Medical Internet Research, 26(4), e51478. https://doi.org/10.2196/51478

Ahola, K., Toppinen-Tanner, S., & Seppänen, J. (2017). Interventions to alleviate burnout symptoms and to support return to work among employees with burnout: Systematic review and meta-analysis. Scandinavian Journal of Work, Environment & Health, 43(4), 293-310.

Ai, W., Cunningham, W. A., & Lai, M. C. (2024). Camouflaging, internalized stigma, and mental health in the general population. Social Psychiatry and Psychiatric Epidemiology, 47(3), 112-128.

Amir, M., Kant, R., & Cheung, L. (2024). A review of psychological resilience: Paving the path for sustainable consumption. Cogent Business & Management, 11(1), 2408436.
https://doi.org/10.1080/23311975.2024.2408436

Appiah, R., Ness, O., & Boakye, K. E. (2024). Editorial: Breaking the mental health stigma for people with substance use disorders. Frontiers in Psychiatry, 15, 1481215.

Babic, A., Lackovic, M., & Stojiljkovic, D. (2022). Post-traumatic growth and psychological resilience during the COVID-19 pandemic: A serial mediation model. Frontiers in Psychiatry, 13, 780807. https://doi.org/10.3389/fpsyt.2022.780807

Bauer, A., Parkinson, S., Startup, H., Broadbent, M., Wheatley, J., Qureshi, A., & Schmidt, U. (2024). The effectiveness of mindfulness-based interventions on anxiety disorders: A systematic meta-review. Clinical Psychology Review, 112, 102314. https://doi.org/10.1016/j.cpr.2024.102314

Bianchi, R., Verkuilen, J., Schonfeld, I. S., Hakanen, J. J., Jansson-Fröjmark, M., Manzano-García, G., ... & Meier, L. L. (2021). Is burnout a depressive condition? A 14-sample meta-analytic and bifactor analytic study. Clinical Psychological Science, 9(4), 579-597.

Branje, S., & de Moor, E. L. (2023). The development of adolescents' loneliness during the COVID-19 pandemic: The role of peer status and contact with friends. PLOS ONE, 18(5), Article e0286046. https://doi.org/10.1371/journal.pone.0286046

Bowden, J. G., Tay, L., Lim, K. W., & Eze, V. N. (2024). What kind of a problem is loneliness? Representations of connectedness and participation from a study of telepresence technologies in the UK. Frontiers in Digital Health, 6, Article 1304085. https://doi.org/10.3389/fdgth.2024.1304085

Cardwell, K., Kerse, N., Hughes, C., Teh, R., Moyes, S., Menzies, O., Rolleston, A., Hayman, K., Wham, C., Jatrana, S., & Kepa, M. (2024). The use of technology to address loneliness and social isolation among older adults: The role of social care providers. BMC Public Health, 24, Article 77. https://doi.org/10.1186/s12889-023-17386-w

Childs, E., & de Wit, H. (2014). Regular exercise is associated with emotional resilience to acute stress in healthy adults. Journal of Health Psychology, 19(6), 734-743. https://doi.org/10.1177/1359105313509965

Corrigan, P. W., & Watson, A. C. (2002). Understanding the impact of stigma on people with mental illness. World Psychiatry, 1(1), 16-20.

Duradoni, M., Collodi, S., Perfumi, S. C., & Guazzini, A. (2024). Exploring the relationships between digital life balance and Internet social capital, loneliness, fear of missing out, and anxiety. Human Behavior and Emerging Technologies, 2024, Article 5079719. https://doi.org/10.1155/2024/5079719

World Health Organization. (2022). Mental health and climate change: Policy brief. WHO Press.

Chang, F., & Lee, C. (2024). Functional connectivity changes in the brain of adolescents with internet addiction: A systematic literature review of imaging studies. PLOS Mental Health, 1(1), e0000022. https://doi.org/10.1371/journal.pmen.0000022

Chen, E. (2024). Neuroplasticity and Anxiety: Rewiring the Brain for Resilience. Stanford Anxiety and Stress Research Center.

Chen, L., Wang, S., Zhang, X., Liu, Y., & Kim, J. (2024). Screen time and mental health: A prospective analysis of the Adolescent Brain Cognitive Development (ABCD) Study. BMC Public Health, 24, 2714. https://doi.org/10.1186/s12889-024-20102-x

Chen, S., Liu, Y., & Zhang, X. (2024). Mindfulness-based stress reduction techniques in educational settings: A new approach to enhance mental health and learning. ResearchGate. https://doi.org/10.13140/RG.2.2.34567.89012

Coronado-Montoya, S., Levis, A. W., Kwakkenbos, L., Steele, R. J., Turner, E. H., & Thombs, B. D. (2024). Reporting of positive results in randomized controlled trials of mindfulness-based mental health interventions. PLOS One, 19(4), e0297714. https://doi.org/10.1371/journal.pone.0297714

Conversano, C., Carbone, G. A., Planned, D., Ciacchini, R., Gemignani, A., & Orrù, G. (2022). Resilience and stress as mediators in the relationship of mindfulness and happiness. Frontiers in Psychology, 13, 771263. https://doi.org/10.3389/fpsyg.2022.771263

De Beer, L. T., Schaufeli, W. B., De Witte, H., Hakanen, J. J., Shimazu, A., Glaser, J., ... & Rudolph, C. W. (2020). Measurement invariance of the burnout assessment tool (BAT) across seven cross-national representative samples.

International Journal of Environmental Research and Public Health, 17(15), 5604.

Dray, J., Bowman, J., Campbell, E., Freund, M., Wolfenden, L., Hodder, R. K., ... & Wiggers, J. (2017). Systematic review of universal resilience-focused interventions targeting child and adolescent mental health in the school setting. Journal of the American Academy of Child & Adolescent Psychiatry, 56(10), 813-824. https://doi.org/10.1016/j.jaac.2017.07.780

Dunning, D., Tudor, K., Radley, L., Dalrymple, N., Funk, J., Vainre, M., ... & Kuyken, W. (2023). Do mindfulness-based programmes improve the cognitive skills, behaviour and mental health of children and adolescents? An updated meta-analysis of randomised controlled trials. Evidence-Based Mental Health, 26(3), 90-98. https://doi.org/10.1136/ebmental-2023-300464

Dweck, C. S. (2016). Mindset: The new psychology of success (Updated edition). Random House.

Erhart, M., Herpertz-Dahlmann, B., Wille, N., Sawitzky-Rose, B., Hölling, H., & Ravens-Sieberer, U. (2018). Examining the relationship between attention-deficit/hyperactivity disorder and overweight in children and adolescents. European Child & Adolescent Psychiatry, 27(4), 493-505. https://doi.org/10.1007/s00787-017-1047-9

Ernst, M., Niederer, D., Werner, A. M., Czaja, S. J., Mikton, C., Ong, A. D., Rosen, T., Brähler, E., & Beutel, M. E. (2022). Loneliness before and during the COVID-19 pandemic: A systematic review with meta-analysis. American Psychologist, 77(5), 660-677.

Fan, X., Chen, P., Zhong, C., Shan, Y., Zhang, J., & Niu, G. (2024). The relationship between loneliness and problematic social media usage in Chinese university students: A longitudinal study. BMC Psychology, 12, Article 10. https://doi.org/10.1186/s40359-023-01498-4

Freudenberger, H. J. (1974). Staff burn-out. Journal of Social Issues, 30(1), 159-165. doi: 10.1111/j.1540-4560.1974.tb00706.x

Fernandes, G. S., Gomes, H. S., Teixeira-Santos, L., Outeiro, T. F., Sousa, N., Pego, J. M., & Summavielle, T. (2024). Exploring the sustained impact of the mindfulness-based stress reduction program: A thematic analysis. Frontiers in Psychology, 15, 1347336. https://doi.org/10.3389/fpsyg.2024.1347336

Fernández-Jiménez, E., & Acquadro Maran, D. (2024). Editorial: Break the mental health stigma: mental health in the workplace. Frontiers in Psychiatry, 15, 1427097.

Fernández-Rodrigues, V., Sanchez-Gonzalez, J., Lahera, G., Diez-Alegria, C., & Montes, J. M. (2024). Current diagnosis and treatment of anxiety disorders. Current Opinion in Psychiatry, 37(2), 125-133. https://doi.org/10.1097/YCO.000000000000

Ferguson, A. M., Cameron, L. D., Deka, P., Wiley, J. F., & Lau-Zhu, A. (2023). The impact of social media use interventions on mental well-being: Systematic review.

Journal of Medical Internet Research, 25, e44922. https://doi.org/10.2196/44922

Ferreira, C., Worthman, C., & Vera-Estay, E. (2024). Digital interventions to promote psychological resilience: A systematic review and meta-analysis. npj Digital Medicine, 7, 34. https://doi.org/10.1038/s41746-024-01017-8

Fu, E., Leung, D. Y. P., Wong, E. M. L., Cheung, D. S. K., & Lam, S. C. (2024). Interventions to reduce loneliness in community-living older adults: A systematic review and meta-analysis. Journal of the American Geriatrics Society, 72(5), 1432-1450.

Galante, J., Friedrich, C., Dawson, A. F., Modrego-Alarcón, M., Gebbing, P., Delgado-Suárez, I., ... & Jones, P. B. (2023). Systematic review and individual participant data meta-analysis of randomized controlled trials assessing mindfulness-based programs for mental health promotion. Nature Mental Health, 1(7), 462-476. https://doi.org/10.1038/s44220-023-00081-5

Ghai, S., Magana, C., Landry, A., & Griffiths, M. D. (2024). Digital detox and well-being: A state-of-the-art review. Current Opinion in Psychology, 59, 101836. https://doi.org/10.1016/j.copsyc.2024.101836

Goleman, D. (2020). Emotional intelligence: Why it matters more than IQ (25th anniversary edition). Bantam Books.

Gyamfi, N., Sukumaran, S., & Kretchy, I. A. (2024). Enablers of mental illness stigma: A scoping review of individual perceptions. Mental Illness, 2024, 8191281.

Halbesleben, J. R., & Buckley, M. R. (2004). Burnout in organizational life. Journal of Management, 30(6), 859-879.

Hawkley, L. C., & Cacioppo, J. T. (2010). Loneliness matters: A theoretical and empirical review of consequences and mechanisms. Annals of Behavioral Medicine, 40(2), 218-227. https://doi.org/10.1007/s12160-010-9210-8

Hayes, S. C., Strosahl, K. D., & Wilson, K. G. (2023). Acceptance and commitment therapy: The process and practice of mindful change (2nd ed.). Journal of Clinical Psychology, 79(4), 812-829. https://doi.org/10.1002/jclp.23456

Helmreich, I., Kunzler, A., Chmitorz, A., König, J., Binder, H., Wessa, M., & Lieb, K. (2017). Psychological interventions for resilience enhancement in adults. Cochrane Database of Systematic Reviews, 2017(2), CD012527. https://doi.org/10.1002/14651858.CD012527

Henderson, C., Noblett, J., Parke, H., Clement, S., Caffrey, A., Gale-Grant, O., .& Thornicroft, G. (2023). Evidence for the effectiveness of interventions to reduce mental health related stigma in the workplace: A systematic review. BMC Psychiatry, 23(1), 184-197.

Hickin, N., Käll, A., Shafran, R., Sutcliffe, S., Manzotti, G., & Langan, D. (2021). The effectiveness of psychological interventions for loneliness: A systematic review and meta-analysis. Clinical Psychology Review, 88, Article 102066. https://doi.org/10.1016/j.cpr.2021.102066

Hoogland, M., & Ploeger, A. (2024). Mismatch resistance and the problem of evolutionary novelty. Biological Theory, 19(3), 123-145. https://doi.org/10.1007/s13752-024-00468-2

Hu, T., Zhang, D., Wang, J., Mistry, R., Ran, G., & Wang, X. (2014). Relation between emotion regulation and mental health: A meta-analysis review. Psychological Reports, 114(2), 341-362. https://doi.org/10.2466/03.20.PR0.114k22w4

Hunt, M. G., Marx, R., Lipson, C., & Young, J. (2022). Effects of limiting digital screen use on well-being, mood, and biomarkers of stress in adults. npj Mental Health Research, 1, 15. https://doi.org/10.1038/s44184-022-00015-6

Hussain, Z., Wegmann, E., Yang, H., Montag, C., & Pontes, H. M. (2024). Impacts of digital social media detox for mental health: A systematic review and meta-analysis. Telemedicine and e-Health, 30(9), 2463-2475. https://doi.org/10.1089/tmj.2024.0106

Hsu, H. C., Chen, L. K., Wu, C. J., Huang, Y. C., Huang, C. C., & Chang, Y. P. (2024). Effectiveness of individual-based strategies to reduce nurse burnout: An umbrella review. Journal of Nursing Management, 32(4), e8544725.

Jin, Y., Sha, S., Tian, T., Wang, Q., Liang, S., Wang, Z., Liu, Y., Cheung, T., Su, Z., & Xiang, Y. T. (2024). How enterprise social media usage links to counterproductive work behavior: The mediating role of workplace loneliness and the moderating role of ICT hassle. Frontiers in Psychology, 15, Article 1328650. https://doi.org/10.3389/fpsyg.2024.1328650

Kabat-Zinn, J. (2019). Wherever you go, there you are: Mindfulness meditation in everyday life (25th anniversary edition). Hachette Books.

Kalisch, R., Baker, D. G., Basten, U., Boks, M. P., Bonanno, G. A., Brummelman, E., ... & Kleim, B. (2017). The resilience framework as a strategy to combat stress-related disorders. Nature Human Behaviour, 1(11), 784-790. https://doi.org/10.1038/s41562-017-0200-8

Kubzansky, L. D., Huffman, J. C., Boehm, J. K., Hernandez, R., Kim, E. S., Koga, H. K., Feig, E. H., Lloyd-Jones, D. M., Seligman, M. E. P., & Labarthe, D. R. (2021). Positive psychological well-being and cardiovascular disease: JACC health promotion series. Circulation Research, 129(8), 1677-1696. https://doi.org/10.1161/CIRCRESAHA.121.319312

Knaak, S., Mantler, E., & Szeto, A. (2017). Mental illness-related stigma in healthcare: Barriers to access and care and evidence-based solutions. Healthcare Management Forum, 30(2), 111-116.

Koutsimani, P., Montgomery, A., & Georganta, K. (2019). The relationship between burnout, depression, and anxiety:

A systematic review and meta-analysis. Frontiers in Psychology, 10, 284.

Lee, R. T., & Ashforth, B. E. (1996). A meta-analytic examination of the correlates of the three dimensions of job burnout. Journal of Applied Psychology, 81(2), 123-133.

Li, N. P., van Vugt, M., & Colarelli, S. M. (2022). Two different mismatches: Integrating the developmental and the evolutionary-mismatch hypothesis. Perspectives on Psychological Science, 17(4), 1025-1040. https://doi.org/10.1177/17456916221078318

Li, Y., & Tang, C. (2024). A systematic review of the effects of rumination-focused cognitive behavioral therapy in reducing depressive symptoms. Frontiers in Psychology, 15, 1447207. https://doi.org/10.3389/fpsyg.2024.1447207

Lim, M. H., Eres, R., & Vasan, S. (2020). Understanding loneliness in the twenty-first century: An update on correlates, risk factors, and potential solutions. Social Psychiatry and Psychiatric Epidemiology, 55(7), 793-810. https://doi.org/10.1007/s00127-020-01889-7

Liu, J. J., Reed, M., & Girard, T. A. (2017). Advancing resilience: An integrative, multi-system model of resilience. Personality and Individual Differences, 111, 111-118. https://doi.org/10.1016/j.paid.2017.02.007

Liu, Y., Zhang, N., Bao, G., Huang, Y., Ji, B., Wu, Y., Liu, C., & Li, G. (2024). Comprehensive review of chronic stress pathways and the efficacy of behavioral stress reduction programs (BSRPs) in managing diseases. International

Journal of Environmental Research and Public Health, 21(8), 1077. https://doi.org/10.3390/ijerph21081077

Lu, F., Wang, Y., Zhang, H., & Liu, M. (2024). The effect of mindfulness-based interventions on reducing stress in future health professionals: A systematic review and meta-analysis of randomized controlled trials. Applied Psychology: Health and Well-Being, 16(2), 245-268. https://doi.org/10.1111/aphw.12472

Mak, A. D. P., Lam, L. C. W., Cuijpers, P., & Chan, W. C. (2024). Efficacy of Internet-based rumination-focused cognitive behavioral therapy and mindfulness-based intervention with guided support in reducing risks of depression and anxiety: A randomized controlled trial. Applied Psychology: Health and Well-Being, 16(2), 892-915. https://doi.org/10.1111/aphw.12512

Masi, C. M., Chen, H. Y., Hawkley, L. C., & Cacioppo, J. T. (2011). A meta-analysis of interventions to reduce loneliness. Personality and Social Psychology Review, 15(3), 219-266. https://doi.org/10.1177/1088868310377394

Maslach, C., & Jackson, S. E. (1981). The measurement of experienced burnout. Journal of Organizational Behavior, 2(2), 99-113.

Masten, A. S., & Motti-Stefanidi, F. (2020). Multisystem resilience for children and youth in disaster: Reflections in the context of COVID-19. Adversity and Resilience Science, 1(2), 95-106. https://doi.org/10.1007/s42844-020-00010-w

Maslach, C., Schaufeli, W. B., & Leiter, M. P. (2001). Job burnout. Annual Review of Psychology, 52(1), 397-422.

Matousian, N., & Otto, K. (2023). How to measure mental illness stigma at work: development and validation of the workplace mental illness stigma scale. Frontiers in Psychiatry, 14, 1225838.

McMillan, S. S., King, M., & Tully, M. P. (2016). How to use the nominal group and Delphi techniques. International Journal of Clinical Pharmacy, 38(3), 655-662. https://doi.org/10.1007/s11096-016-0257-x

Mehta, N., Clement, S., Marcus, E., Stona, A. C., Bezborodovs, N., Evans-Lacko, S., ... & Thornicroft, G. (2015). Evidence for effective interventions to reduce mental health-related stigma and discrimination in the medium and long term: Systematic review. British Journal of Psychiatry, 207(5), 377-384.

Melumad, S., Inman, J. J., & Pham, M. T. (2023). Taking a break: The effects of partaking in a two-week social media digital detox on problematic smartphone and social media use, and other health-related outcomes among young adults. Cyberpsychology, Behavior, and Social Networking, 26(12), 907-916. https://doi.org/10.1089/cyber.2023.0049

Mihalopoulos, C., Le, L. K. D., Chatterton, M. L., Bucholc, J., Holt-Lunstad, J., Lim, M. H., & Engel, L. (2020). The economic costs of loneliness: A review of cost-of-illness and economic evaluation studies. Social Psychiatry and Psychiatric Epidemiology, 55(7), 823-836. https://doi.org/10.1007/s00127-019-01733-7

Modrego-Alarcón, M., Margolles, R., González-García, P., Ruiz-Robledillo, N., Santed, M. A., Pérez-Yus, M. C., ... & García-Campayo, J. (2021). Mindfulness-based programmes for mental health promotion in adults in nonclinical settings: A systematic review and meta-analysis of randomised controlled trials. PLOS Medicine, 18(1), e1003481. https://doi.org/10.1371/journal.pmed.1003481

Mueller, C., Jaud, S., Wertli, M., Glinz, D., Zeller, A., Hemkens, L. G., & Tal, K. (2024). The interplay of stress, health, and well-being: Unraveling the psychological and physiological processes. Frontiers in Psychology, 15, 1471084. https://doi.org/10.3389/fpsyg.2024.1471084

Neff, K. (2019). Self-compassion: The proven power of being kind to yourself. William Morrow Paperbacks.

Park, C., Majeed, A., Gill, H., Tamura, J., Ho, R. C., Mansur, R. B., Nasri, F., Lee, Y., Rosenblat, J. D., Wong, E., & McIntyre, R. S. (2020). The effect of loneliness on distinct health outcomes: A comprehensive review and meta-analysis. Psychiatry Research, 294, Article 113514. https://doi.org/10.1016/j.psychres.2020.113514

Pertl, M. T., Robertson, D. A., Walsh, C., Horan, E., Keogh, A., Finn, C., McCrory, C., & Kenny, R. A. (2023). Understanding loneliness in younger people: Review of the opportunities and challenges for loneliness interventions. Interactive Journal of Medical Research, 12, Article e45197. https://doi.org/10.2196/45197

Prime, H., Wade, M., & Browne, D. T. (2020). Risk and resilience in family well-being during the COVID-19 pandemic. American Psychologist, 75(5), 631-643. https://doi.org/10.1037/amp0000660

Puolakanaho, A., Tolvanen, A., Kinnunen, S. M., & Lappalainen, R. (2022). Mindfulness-based online intervention increases well-being and decreases stress after Covid-19 lockdown. Scientific Reports, 12, 6562. https://doi.org/10.1038/s41598-022-10361-2

Radtke, T., Apel, T., Schenkel, K., Keller, J., & von Lindern, E. (2025). Digital detox strategies and mental health: A comprehensive scoping review of why, where, and how. Cureus, 17(1), e74521. https://doi.org/10.7759/cureus.74521

Reangsing, C., Rittiwong, T., & Schneider, J. K. (2021). Effects of mindfulness meditation interventions on depression, anxiety, and psychological well-being in older adults: A systematic review. Journal of Geriatric Psychiatry and Neurology, 34(3), 181-200. https://doi.org/10.1177/0891988720967303

Richman, L. S., Kubzansky, L., Maselko, J., Kawachi, I., Choo, P., & Bauer, M. (2005). Positive emotion and health: Going beyond the negative. Health Psychology, 24(4), 422-429. https://doi.org/10.1037/0278-6133.24.4.422

Rodrigues, M. F., Nardi, A. E., & Levitan, M. (2017). Mindfulness in mood and anxiety disorders: A review of the literature. Trends in Psychiatry and Psychotherapy, 39(3), 207-215. https://doi.org/10.1590/2237-6089-2016-0051

Rogers, A. A., Ha, T., & Ockey, S. (2021). Adolescents' perceived socio-emotional impact of COVID-19 and implications for mental health: Results from a U.S.-based mixed-methods study. Journal of Adolescent Health, 68(1), 43-52. https://doi.org/10.1016/j.jadohealth.2020.09.039

Salvagioni, D. A. J., Melanda, F. N., Mesas, A. E., González, A. D., Gabani, F. L., & Andrade, S. M. D. (2017). Physical, psychological and occupational consequences of job burnout: A systematic review of prospective studies. PLoS One, 12(10), e0185781.

Saritepeci, M., & Çakır, H. (2023). The effects of digital addiction on brain function and structure of children and adolescents: A scoping review. Healthcare, 12(1), 15. https://doi.org/10.3390/healthcare12010015

Sarris, J., Camfield, D., & Berk, M. (2012). Complementary medicine, self-help, and lifestyle interventions for anxiety disorders. Australian & New Zealand Journal of Psychiatry, 46(9), 813-828. https://doi.org/10.1177/0004867412444400

Seligman, M. E. P. (2018). Learned optimism: How to change your mind and your life (Vintage Books edition). Vintage Books.

Sexton, M. B., Hamilton, L., McGinnis, E. W., Rosenblum, K. L., & Muzik, M. (2015). The roles of resilience and childhood trauma history: Main and moderating effects on postpartum maternal mental health and functioning. Journal of Affective Disorders, 174, 562-568. https://doi.org/10.1016/j.jad.2014.12.036

Sood, A., Prasad, K., Schroeder, D., & Varkey, P. (2011). Stress management and resilience training among Department of Medicine faculty: A pilot randomized clinical trial. Journal of General Internal Medicine, 26(8), 858-861. https://doi.org/10.1007/s11606-011-1640-x

Southwick, S. M., Bonanno, G. A., Masten, A. S., Panter-Brick, C., & Yehuda, R. (2014). Resilience definitions, theory, and challenges: Interdisciplinary perspectives. European Journal of Psychotraumatology, 5(1), 25338. https://doi.org/10.3402/ejpt.v5.25338

Shah, S. G. S., Nogueras, D., van Woerden, H. C., & Kiparoglou, V. (2020). Loneliness and social isolation interventions for older adults: A scoping review of reviews. BMC Public Health, 20, Article 129. https://doi.org/10.1186/s12889-020-8251-6

Stiglic, N., & Viner, R. M. (2021). The relationship between screen time and mental health in young people: A systematic review of longitudinal studies. Clinical Psychology Review, 86, 102021. https://doi.org/10.1016/j.cpr.2021.102021

Strauss, C., Cavanagh, K., Oliver, A., & Pettman, D. (2014). Mindfulness-based interventions for people diagnosed with a current episode of an anxiety or depressive disorder: A meta-analysis of randomised controlled trials. PLOS One, 9(4), e96110. https://doi.org/10.1371/journal.pone.0096110

Stockings, E. A., Degenhardt, L., Dobbins, T., Lee, Y. Y., Erskine, H. E., Whiteford, H. A., & Patton, G. (2016).

Preventing depression and anxiety in young people: A review of the joint efficacy of universal, selective, and indicated prevention. Psychological Medicine, 46(1), 11-26. https://doi.org/10.1017/S0033291715001725

Lizano, E. L., Hsiao, H. Y., Mor Barak, M. E., & Casper, L. M. (2014). Support in the workplace: Buffering the deleterious effects of work–family conflict on child welfare workers' well-being and job burnout. Health & Social Work, 39(1), 55-65. doi:10.1093/hsw/hlu007

Shin, J., Lee, Y., Oh, K. S., Kim, M., Jung, S., Shin, A., ... & Kim, M. (2023). Neuropsychology of generalized anxiety disorder in clinical setting: A systematic evaluation. Healthcare, 11(17), 2446. https://doi.org/10.3390/healthcare11172446

Subu, M. A., Holmes, D., Elliot, R., & Martyn, H. (2021). Types of stigma experienced by patients with mental illness and mental health nurses in Indonesia: A qualitative content analysis. International Journal of Mental Health Systems, 15(1), 1-12.

Surkalim, D. L., Luo, M., Eres, R., Gebel, K., van Busschbach, J., Bauman, A., & Ding, D. (2022). The prevalence of loneliness across 113 countries: Systematic review and meta-analysis. BMJ, 376, Article e067068. https://doi.org/10.1136/bmj-2021-067068

Sutherland, R., Yap, M. B. H., Youssef, G. J., Pennell, K., Lubman, D. I., Masson, V. L., ... & Olsson, C. A. (2019). A longitudinal study of the adolescent risk-mental health paradox. Journal of Clinical Child & Adolescent

Psychology, 48(2), 290-302. https://doi.org/10.1080/15374416.2018.1421516

Tedeschi, R. G., Shakespeare-Finch, J., Taku, K., & Calhoun, L. G. (2018). Posttraumatic growth: Theory, research, and applications. Routledge.

Thoma, M. V., Rohleder, N., & Rohner, S. L. (2023). Mindfulness training, cognitive performance and stress reduction: Evidence from a randomized controlled trial. Journal of Economic Behavior & Organization, 214, 512-535. https://doi.org/10.1016/j.jebo.2023.10.008

Thompson, A., Hunt, C., & Issakidis, C. (2004). Why wait? Reasons for delay and prompts to seek help for mental health problems in an Australian clinical sample. Social Psychiatry and Psychiatric Epidemiology, 39(10), 810-817.

Throuvala, M. A., Janikian, M., Griffiths, M. D., Rennoldson, M., & Kuss, D. J. (2023). A comprehensive review on emerging trends in the dynamic evolution of digital addiction and depression. Frontiers in Psychology, 14, 1126815. https://doi.org/10.3389/fpsyg.2023.1126815

Twenge, J. M., & Campbell, W. K. (2018). Associations between screen time and lower psychological well-being among children and adolescents: Evidence from a population-based study. Preventive Medicine, 112, 271-283. https://doi.org/10.1016/j.ypmed.2018.04.011

Unützer, J., Kimmel, R. J., & Snowden, M. (2016). Psychiatry in the age of neuroscience and genome-wide association studies. The Lancet Psychiatry, 3(2), 179-186.

U.S. Department of Health and Human Services. (2023). Our epidemic of loneliness and isolation: The U.S. Surgeon General's advisory on the healing effects of social connection and community. Office of the Surgeon General.

Vaillant, G. E. (2012). Triumphs of experience: The men of the Harvard Grant Study. Little, Brown and Company.

van Vugt, M., Colarelli, S. M., & Li, N. P. (2024). Digitally connected, evolutionarily wired: An evolutionary mismatch perspective on digital work. Evolutionary Psychology, 22(1). https://doi.org/10.1177/20413866241232138

van Winkel, M., Wichers, M., Collip, D., Jacobs, N., Derom, C., Thiery, E., Myin-Germeys, I., & Peeters, F. (2017). Unraveling the role of loneliness in depression: The relationship between daily life experience and behavior. Psychiatry Research, 252, 262-268. https://doi.org/10.1016/j.psychres.2017.03.021

Vaillant, G. E. (2012). Triumphs of experience: The men of the Harvard Grant Study. Little, Brown and Company.

Vøllestad, J., Nielsen, M. B., & Nielsen, G. H. (2012). Mindfulness- and acceptance-based interventions for anxiety disorders: A systematic review and meta-analysis. British Journal of Clinical Psychology, 51(3), 239-260. https://doi.org/10.1111/j.2044-8260.2011.02024.x

White, B., Clark, A., & Miller, M. (2024). Digital being: Social media and the predictive mind. Neuroscience of Consciousness, 2024(1), niae008. https://doi.org/10.1093/nc/niae008

Weil, A. (2020). Breathing: The master key to self healing. Sounds True Publishing.

West, C. P., Dyrbye, L. N., & Shanafelt, T. D. (2018). Physician burnout: Contributors, consequences, and solutions. Journal of Internal Medicine, 283(6), 516-529.

Windle, G. (2011). What is resilience? A review and concept analysis. Reviews in Clinical Gerontology, 21(2), 152-169. https://doi.org/10.1017/S0959259810000420

World Health Organization. (2019). Burn-out an "occupational phenomenon": International Classification of Diseases. ICD-11 for Mortality and Morbidity Statistics. Geneva: World Health Organization.

World Health Organization. (2022). Mental health and climate change: Policy brief. Geneva: World Health Organization Press.

Yanos, P. T., Lucksted, A., Drapalski, A. L., Roe, D., & Lysaker, P. (2015). Interventions targeting mental health self-stigma: A review and comparison. Psychiatric Rehabilitation Journal, 38(2), 171-178.

Yim, O. S. (2023). The Internet and loneliness. AMA Journal of Ethics, 25(11), E850-E856. https://doi.org/10.1001/amajethics.2023.850

Young, K. S., Sandman, C. F., & Craske, M. G. (2019). Positive and negative emotion regulation in adolescence: Links to anxiety and depression. Brain Sciences, 9(4), 76. https://doi.org/10.3390/brainsci9040076

Youssef-Morgan, C. M., & Luthans, F. (2015). Psychological capital and well-being. Stress and Health, 31(3), 180-188. https://doi.org/10.1002/smi.2623

Joyce, S., Shand, F., Tighe, J., Laurent, S. J., Bryant, R. A., & Harvey, S. B. (2018). Road to resilience: A systematic review and meta-analysis of resilience training programmes and interventions. BMJ Open, 8(6), e017858. https://doi.org/10.1136/bmjopen-2017-017858

Zeng, P., & Hu, X. (2024). A study of the psychological mechanisms of job burnout: Implications of person–job fit and person–organization fit. Frontiers in Psychology, 15, 1351032.

Zhang, M., Murphy, B., Cabaniss, W., & Yidi, C. (2022). The study of mindfulness as an intervening factor for enhanced psychological well-being in building the level of resilience. Frontiers in Psychology, 13, 1056834. https://doi.org/10.3389/fpsyg.2022.1056834

Zhou, X., Guo, J., Lu, G., Chen, C., Xie, Z., Liu, J., & Zhang, C. (2023). Effects of mindfulness-based interventions on stress and burnout in nurses: A systematic review and meta-analysis. Frontiers in Psychiatry, 14, 1029582. https://doi.org/10.3389/fpsyt.2023.1029582

About the Author

Clara Solace is an author, emotional wellness advocate, and passionate mental health supporter. With deep empathy for everyday struggles, she empowers readers with simple yet meaningful strategies for navigating life's challenges.

She believes in the power of stillness, resilience, and intentional living. Her work offers gentle guidance and hope to anyone feeling overwhelmed in today's fast paced world.

When she's not writing, Clara enjoys creating uplifting content, encouraging others through heartfelt conversations, and exploring ways to bring more peace and purpose into daily life.

Connect with her:

Email: clarasolace.author@gmail.com

www.ingramcontent.com/pod-product-compliance
Lightning Source LLC
LaVergne TN
LVHW100728061126
851857LV00011B/443
9783982782423